THE PHARMACIST'S GU

Evidence-Based Medicine

for Clinical Decision Making

Patrick J. Bryant, Pharm.D., FSCIP

Director, Drug Information Center
Clinical Professor, Pharmacy Practice
University of Missouri–Kansas City School
of Pharmacy
Kansas City, Missouri

Heather A. Pace, Pharm.D.

Assistant Director, Drug Information Center
Clinical Assistant Professor, Pharmacy Practice
University of Missouri–Kansas City School
of Pharmacy
Kansas City, Missouri

American Society of Health-System Pharmacists®
Bethesda, Maryland

Director, Special Publishing: Jack Bruggeman
Acquisitions Editor: Hal Pollard
Senior Editorial Project Manager: Dana Battaglia
Project Editor: Johnna Hershey
Cover and Page Design/Composition: David A. Wade

Library of Congress Cataloging-in-Publication Data

Bryant, Patrick J.
  The pharmacist's guide to evidence-based medicine for clinical decision making / Patrick J. Bryant, Heather A. Pace.
      p. ; cm.
  Includes bibliographical references and index.
  ISBN 978-1-58528-177-0
  1. Pharmacy--Decision making. 2. Evidence-based medicine. I. Pace, Heather A. II. American Society of Health-System Pharmacists. III. Title.
  [DNLM: 1. Drug Therapy. 2. Decision Making. 3. Evidence-Based Medicine. 4. Pharmacology, Clinical. WB 330 B915p 2008]

  RS92.B765 2008
  615'.1--dc22
                                    2008034439

Table of Contents

Acknowledgments

The development of a unique process like the one described in this book is not an easy task and has involved many different minds over several years. We would like to thank those residents and fellows that have trained in the University of Missouri–Kansas City School of Pharmacy Drug Information Center for their assistance and feedback used to modify and improve the process.

These people include Antoine Richardson (also previous faculty), Jessica Beal, Michael Steinberg, Julie Kenkel, Kevin Clauson, Kelly Shields, Marissa Curiel-Dickson, Elizabeth Poole, Celtina Reinert, and Melita Croom. We would also like to thank those drug information faculty who have made contributions to the process, including Cydney McQueen (also previous Fellow), Lindsey Schnabel (also previous Resident), Morgan Sperry, Karen Norris, Angela Bedenbaugh, and Chris Meier.

Denise Woolf with our Center has been monumental in proofreading and suggesting changes that make the book more readable and understandable; we thank her for this contribution.

Over 600 students have passed through the evidence-based medicine course and provided feedback to improve this process. Specifically, we want to thank Amber Sawyer for reading through the book and identifying evidence-based medicine terms for the glossary from a student's perspective.

Tim Candy, Manager, Global Medical/Clinical Affairs at Baxter Healthcare Corporation, deserves a huge thank you for his contributions to the Basics for Interpretation chapter. He was also responsible for providing the biostatistics section of the Evidence-Based Medicine Glossary. We also thank Seth Berry, Associate Director, Modeling and Simulation at Quintiles, Inc., for his help with the Basics for Interpretation chapter.

We would like to thank our Pharmacy Practice Faculty colleagues for their curb-side consults as we developed this process. Specifically, we thank Brooke Patterson, Jennifer Santee, and

Tatum Mead for reviewing the chapter on Basics for Interpretation and providing feedback on the clarity and ease of reading this section of the book.

This project would never have happened without Hal Pollard, Content Development & Acquisitions Editor at the American Society of Health-System Pharmacists (ASHP), who caught and supported our vision for a "how to" book on this subject. We thank you Hal for your continued encouragement and support throughout this project. We would also like to thank Jack Bruggeman, Director, ASHP's Special Publishing, for providing the resources to see this project through. We now have a better appreciation for the job that Dana Battaglia, Senior Editorial Project Manager at ASHP, does; she gets a special thank you for training us to be book editors, not to mention the long hours she spent reviewing and providing feedback for our multiple drafts. Johnna Hershey, Director, ASHP's Publications Production Center in the Publications and Drug Information Systems Office, certainly deserves a big thank you for her copy editing and final production work with this book. A thanks goes out to all those at ASHP who have played some part in the development and production of this book.

No project of this magnitude happens without the administrative support provided by the Chair of Pharmacy Practice, Patricia Marken and Dean Robert Piepho. Thank you both for your patience and guidance.

Perhaps most important is our thanks to each of our families for their encouragement and patience while we took time away from them to work on this project. They have played such a key role in allowing this project to be completed.

Pat Bryant

Heather Pace

Preface

Evidence-based medicine has been taught in a focused manner at the University of Missouri–Kansas City School of Pharmacy since 1998. Over that time, a unique systematic approach has been developed that caters to the analytical mind of the pharmacy practitioner. This book represents an attempt to transfer this process to pharmacy students and practitioners for maximizing clinical decision making.

Other evidence-based medicine processes have proven to be complex, labor intensive, and time consuming. The *5-Step Evidence-Based Process* described in this book comes out of simplifying the complexity while still maintaining adequate rigor. This allows the practitioner to apply the process to every day, individual patient and population-based, time sensitive decision making.

This is a "how to" book not a text book, although we anticipate the book will be a valuable addition to literature evaluation, evidence-based medicine, and drug information courses. The book was especially developed for the busy practitioner who can read through the text in an evening or two and immediately apply the *5-Step Evidence-Based Medicine Process* to his or her practice setting. Although there is an assumed minimal level of pharmacotherapy, literature evaluation, study design, and interpretive biostatistics knowledge for the reader, reference to additional reading is made to assist those requiring a review of these foundational topics.

The book is arranged in three specific sections that include an introduction and review of basic study interpretation skills, the specific *5-Step Evidence-Based Medicine Process,* and application of this process to specific individual patient and population-based situations. Think of the book as containing core knowledge based on the *5-Step Evidence-Based Medicine Process* (one chapter for each step). In addition, chapters have been added that will provide the required skills, resources, and examples to put this process into practice.

A seasoned practitioner may want to go directly to those chapters describing the *5-Step Evidence-Based Process*, referring to the other chapters as needed. Other readers are encouraged to read the book from cover to cover, keeping in mind that the book was written and formatted with the intention to be an easy read. Throughout the book, "Key Ideas" are extracted and set out from the text. They serve as a quick review as well as reference points to find specific sections of the text to refer back to as the process is applied in clinical practice. In addition, figures and tables have been used extensively to visually convey concepts. Examples have been provided to illustrate application of these concepts. A Glossary of Evidence-Based Medicine terms has been included at the end of the book to help the reader become familiar with the unique vocabulary associated with this discipline. An Evidence-Based Medicine Tool Kit has also been provided to assist with the initial application of this process to clinical practice.

Our goal is to provide this *5-Step Evidence-Based Medicine Process* to every pharmacy practitioner and student so they can quickly learn and incorporate this process into their clinical decision making. Our hope is that the application of this process to clinical practice will result in overall improved patient care.

Pat Bryant

Heather Pace

Contributors

Patrick J. Bryant, Pharm.D., FSCIP

Director, Drug Information Center
Clinical Professor, Pharmacy Practice
University of Missouri–Kansas City School of Pharmacy
Kansas City, Missouri

Timothy A. Candy, Pharm.D., M.S., BCPS

Manager, Global Medical/Clinical Affairs
Baxter Healthcare Corporation
Round Lake, Illinois

Cydney E. McQueen, Pharm.D.

Clinical Associate Professor, Pharmacy Practice
University of Missouri–Kansas City School of Pharmacy
Kansas City, Missouri

Heather A. Pace, Pharm.D.

Assistant Director, Drug Information Center
Clinical Assistant Professor, Pharmacy Practice
University of Missouri–Kansas City School of Pharmacy
Kansas City, Missouri

Celtina K. Reinert, Pharm.D.

Integrative Therapies Pharmacist
Sastun Center of Integrative Health Care
Overland Park, Kansas

Antoine D. Richardson, Pharm.D.

Clinical Instructor
University of Missouri–Kansas City School of Pharmacy
Kansas City, Missouri

Lindsey N. Schnabel, Pharm.D.

Clinical Assistant Professor, Pharmacy Practice
Assistant Director, Drug Information Center
University of Missouri–Kansas City School of Pharmacy
Kansas City, Missouri

Morgan L. Sperry, Pharm.D.

Clinical Assistant Professor, Pharmacy Practice
Assistant Director, Drug Information Center
University of Missouri–Kansas City School of Pharmacy
Kansas City, Missouri

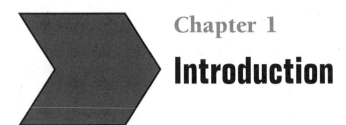

Chapter 1
Introduction

Patrick J. Bryant

Evidence-Based Medicine

Evidence-based medicine focuses on the scientific method as the key source of knowledge in making clinical decisions. Research shows that when we use experience as the primary knowledge source to make clinical decisions, we tend to overestimate efficacy and underestimate risk factors of a specific drug or procedure.[1] This leads to variation in services and treatment, resulting in inappropriate care, lack of care, and increase in health care costs. An approach to making clinical decisions has emerged within the medical discipline called evidence-based medicine. Evidence-based medicine is an attempt to provide something other than just experience of the practitioner in making clinical decisions. David Sackett, one of the pioneers in this area, originally coined the term "evidence-based medicine" while teaching medical students; he essentially defined this term as:

> "The conscientious, explicit, and judicious use of current best evidence in making decisions about the care of individual patients, while integrating clinical experience with the best available evidence from a systematic search."[2]

1

Sources of Knowledge

As mentioned, evidence-based medicine utilizes the scientific method as a key source of knowledge for clinical decision making. However, in addition to the scientific method, there are four other sources of knowledge.[3] Each source or method presents potential problems that are discussed below.

Key Idea

Evidence-based medicine focuses on scientific method as the key source of knowledge to make clinical decisions.

1. **Reference to tradition** – accepting certain truths as givens. Problem: many traditions are not evaluated for validity nor tested against potentially superior alternatives.

2. **Reference to authority** – placing trust in those who are authorities or experts on an issue. This can be useful where scientific evidence is weak or unavailable. Problem: this method minimizes the need for critical analysis and confirmation of validity and does not encourage testing of potentially superior alternatives.

3. **Trial and error** – applying multiple attempts to find a solution by chance. Used when no other basis for making a decision exists. Problem: this method results in a haphazard and unsystematic process to obtain knowledge that is generally not shared, limited in scope, and time consuming; it also prevents identifying/confirming the best solution.

4. **Logical reasoning** – involving *deductive reasoning*—a systematic method for drawing conclusions by using a series of three interrelated statements. Problem: deductive reasoning only produces a hypothesis that still requires testing since usefulness is dependent upon the truth of the premises developed. **Example**—all living things must die (major premise), humans are living things (minor

premise); therefore, all humans must die (conclusion). Logical reasoning also involves *inductive reasoning* or developing generalizations from specific observations. Problem: quality of the knowledge derived from inductive reasoning is dependent upon how well specific observations represent the general situation. To be absolutely certain of the conclusion, one must observe all possible examples of the event, and that is rarely possible. **Example**—edema decreases with application of ice to an injured ankle. After numerous observations of this phenomenon, one concludes cold reduces fluid infiltration in body tissues.

5. **Scientific method** – applying a logical sequential process to develop a conclusion. This process involves identifying the problem, organizing collection of data, objectively analyzing the data, and interpreting the findings. The goal is to enable other researchers to reproduce the results that confirm validity. This is the most rigorous process for obtaining new knowledge. Problem: complexity and variability of components (e.g., nature/environment, unique psychosocial and physiological capacities of individuals) introduce uncertainty into interpretation and generalization of data.

The Problem

Although the best evidence comes from the scientific method, medical practice continues to focus on the other four sources of knowledge. The result is variation in medical practice patterns and variation in treatment for virtually the same patient with the same disease state.[4] In addition, a gap exists between new research findings and incorporating these findings into clinical practice.

Key Idea

Although the best evidence comes from the scientific method, medical practice continues to focus on less accurate sources of knowledge.

As a result, the most recent scientifically developed knowledge is not being applied to clinical practice. The scientific method, our best source of knowledge, is not being maximized to ensure the best patient care.

Several evidence-based medicine processes have been developed; however, these processes tend to be complex, labor intensive, inconsistent in rigor, and variable in determining the quality of evidence. Morever, these processes are generally developed by physicians for diagnostic minded physicians and not for the analytically minded pharmacy practitioner. These practitioners need a time-sensitive decision making process that allows them to make *firm* decisions and recommendations based on results of rigorously conducted clinical trials while incorporating their own clinical judgment. **Figure 1.1** illustrates how the practitioner must use caution in developing a recommendation and/or decision when this type of evidence does not exist.

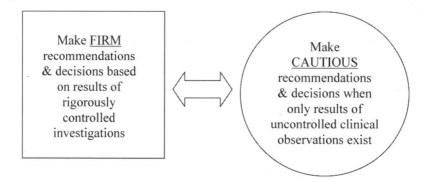

Figure 1.1: Explanation of Differences in Firm and Cautious Recommendations Based on Trial Type

Key Idea

Practitioners need a time-sensitive decision making process that leads to evidence-supported decisions and recommendations.

The Solution

The University of Missouri–Kansas City School of Pharmacy Drug Information Center developed the 5-Step Evidence-Based Medicine Process that has been taught as a required course to Doctor of Pharmacy (Pharm.D.) students for the last 10 years. This process exhibits the following characteristics:

❑ Offers less complexity

❑ Offers time-sensitive decision making support by alleviating time-intensive methods

❑ Maintains rigor

❑ Categorizes quality of the evidence in a simple, straightforward, and logical manner

❑ Provides a process designed specifically for pharmacy practitioners making drug therapy decisions

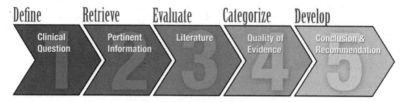

Figure 1.2: 5-Step Evidence-Based Medicine Process

This process involves five steps as illustrated in **Figure 1.2. Step one** is defining the clinical question. Defining the clinical question is essential in providing direction to the remaining four steps of this evidence-based medicine process. This step may be the hardest one in the process because it involves the conversion of a clinical problem into an answerable clinical question. A well-constructed answerable clinical question clearly presents the true clinical problem, provides guidance to pertinent evidence, and suggests the format of the recommendation to solve the problem.

Step two involves searching the literature for articles associated with this clinical question. The assumption is that the reader has completed a basic literature retrieval course. A comprehensive discussion of resources for searching the literature is beyond the scope of this book. Furthermore, most practitioners are too busy to conduct extensive and sophisticated database searches to ensure a comprehensive review of the pertinent literature. For this reason, the practitioner must rely on specialists in drug information centers and health system libraries to conduct the searches for them. Specific references will be identified for readers who want a review of searching processes.

Step three is evaluating literature found. Again, the assumption is that the reader has completed at least a basic critical evaluation course with some exposure to biostatistics. Although it is not a requirement to understand the evidence-based medicine process presented in this book, those readers without this background or those desiring a "refresher" review can refer to additional resources identified throughout the book.

Step four is determining the quality of identified and critically evaluated evidence. Several different hierarchies of evidence are available to accomplish this step.[5–15] The categorization system presented in this book provides a simple, straightforward, and logical approach, which incorporates a modified technique to determine the quality of evidence originally described in Drs. Deborah Cook and Gordon Guyatt's 1992 seminal work.[1] This fourth step serves as a bridge to the fifth step.

Step five is developing a conclusion and recommendation with supporting justification. This step involves the creation of a specific recommendation statement supported by the efficacy, safety, and other special considerations/special populations provided by the evidence. Cost of therapy is also factored into this final recommendation.

How This Book Will Help You

This book is not a text book, but rather a "how to" or self-development type resource. The book teaches the practitioner how to incorporate the 5-Step Evidence-Based Medicine Process into daily drug therapy decision making.

Key Idea	*This book is not a text book, but rather a "how to" or self-development type resource.*

A consistent goal has been to develop an evidence-based medicine process that is simple enough to integrate into practitoners' thought processes without giving up any rigor or quality associated with good clinical decision making. Based on results of studies to determine the effectiveness of this process, this goal has been accomplished over the last 9 years of development.[16] Now, that same evidence-based medicine process is made available to the practitioner through this book.

The format has been carefully considered, allowing the reader to complete the book within a couple of evenings and immediately incorporate the process into current clinical practice. In addition, the reader is encouraged to use this book as a resource while applying the 5-Step Evidence-Based Medicine Process in practice.

Key Idea	*The format allows the reader to complete the book in a couple of evenings and immediately incorporate the process into current clinical practice.*

Chapter 2: Basics for Interpretation is a high-level review of basic tools and concepts associated with study design and selected biostatistic principles. Emphasis is placed specifically on the more pertinent knowledge in these two areas that is required to understand and effectively perform the Evidence-Based Medicine Process. For instance, only four biostatistic concepts are discussed:

1. Significance
2. Power

3. Types of data

4. Appropriate statistical tests for the type of data undergoing analysis

For a more comprehensive review of biostatistics, the reader should refer to the suggested references.

The actual 5-Step Evidence-Based Medicine Process is described in Chapters 3 through 7. Each chapter addresses a specific step in the process. Examples are provided to further illustrate the concepts being taught. In addition, figures and tables are included to reinforce visual learning of the concepts.

Key Idea

The actual 5-Step Evidence-Based Medicine Process is described in Chapters 3 through 7 with each chapter addressing a specific step in the process.

Chapters 8–10 identify special considerations and describe clinical pharmacy practice applications for this process. Chapter 10 has been devoted to the differences in practicing evidence-based medicine with dietary supplements compared to conventional pharmaceuticals. The use of evidence-based medicine practice with dietary supplements is an area requiring greater attention. This chapter is an attempt to address that need.

At the end of this book, you will find a glossary of evidence-based medicine terms to assist in learning the language associated with this discipline. In addition, there is a section dedicated to forms and tables used by our students during the initial stages of learning the 5-Step Evidence-Based Medicine Process. This section is appropriately named Evidence-Based Medicine Tools and will hopefully be a help.

References

1. Cook DJ, Guyatt GH, Laupacis A, et al. Rules of evidence and clinical recommendations on the use of antithrombotic agents. *Chest.* 1992; 102(4 suppl):305S–311S.

2. Sackett DL, Rosenberg WC, Gray JAM, et al. Evidence-based medicine: what it is and what it isn't. *BMJ.* 1996; 312:71–72.

3. Portney LG, Watkins MP. *Foundations of Clinical Research: Applications to Practice.* 2nd ed. Stamford, CT: Appleton & Lange; 2000.

4. Eddy DM. Evidence-based medicine: a unified approach. *Health Affairs.* 2005; 24(1):9–17.

5. Guyatt GH, Sackett DL, Sinclair JC, et al. Users' guides to the medical literature. IX. A method for grading health care recommendations. Evidence-Based Medicine Working Group [published erratum appears in *JAMA.* 1996; 275(16):1232]. *JAMA.* 1995; 274:1800–1804.

6. McGovern DPB, Summerskill WSM, Valori RM, et al. *Key Topics in Evidence-Based Medicine.* Oxford, UK: BIOS Scientific Publishers Limited; 2001.

7. Heneghan C, Badenoch D. *Evidence-based Medicine Toolkit.* Oxford, UK: Blackwell Publishing Limited; 2006.

8. Mayer D. *Essential Evidence-Based Medicine.* Cambridge, UK: Cambridge University Press; 2004.

9. U.S. Preventive Services Task Force. *Guide to Clinical Preventive Services.* 2nd ed. Baltimore, MD: Williams & Wilkins; 1996.

10. The Canadian Task Force on the Periodic Health Examination. *The Canadian Guide to Clinical Preventive Health Care.* Ottawa: Health Canada; 1994.

11. Sackett DL. Rules of evidence and clinical recommendations. *Can J Cardiol.* 1993; 9:487–489.

12. Guyatt G, Rennie D, eds. *User's Guides to the Medical Literature*. Chicago, IL: AMA Press; 2002.

13. Agency for Healthcare Research and Quality. Systems to rate the strength of scientific evidence. Available at: http://www.ahrq.gov/clinic/epcsums/strengthsum.pdf. Accessed April 6, 2007.

14. Scottish Intercollegiate Guidelines Network. SIGN 50: a guideline developer's handbook. Available at: http://www.sign.ac.uk/guidelines/fulltext/50/section6.html. Accessed April 6, 2007.

15. National Institute for Health and Clinical Excellence. Guideline development methods – Chapter 7: reviewing and grading the evidence (revised March 14, 2005). Available at: http://www.nice.org.uk/page.aspx?o=247836. Accessed April 6, 2007.

16. Pace HA, Norris KP, Bryant PJ. Evaluation of evidence-based medicine education at the University of Missouri–Kansas City School of Pharmacy. Unpublished data presented in poster format at the American Association of Colleges of Pharmacy 2006 Annual Meeting in San Diego, CA.

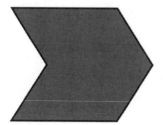

Chapter 2

Basics for Interpretation

Patrick J. Bryant, Heather A. Pace, Timothy A. Candy, & Antoine D. Richardson

Why Should I Read This?

An understanding of some basic study design and statistical concepts is necessary to effectively apply the 5-Step Evidence-Based Medicine Process described in this book. This chapter is not intended to be a comprehensive review of study design and biostatistics. Rather than focusing on selecting and performing specific study designs and statistical tests, this chapter describes practical applications of basic concepts in these two areas with an emphasis on interpretation of clinical research results. For those practitioners who want a full review of either subject, the references used for this chapter provide an excellent list of resources.[1-13] In addition, a glossary of terms frequently used in clinical research articles is provided in the Glossary of Evidence-Based Medicine Terms found in the back of this book.

Essential Study Design Concepts

Interventional Trial Design

An interventional study design, the most familiar study type, is referred to as experimental study design. In this design, subjects receive a treatment (or intervention) they would not otherwise receive, and then the effect on a particular outcome is observed. Subjects are randomly assigned to treatment groups by a randomization scheme. If done correctly, subjects have an equal chance of being assigned to a particular treatment group. All interventional studies are prospective—that is, they look forward in time. Interventional study designs are better at establishing cause-and-effect relationships than observational designs because the influence of confounding factors can be more controlled in an interventional study.

Interventional studies can be either parallel or crossover design. In a parallel design, both groups are given treatment simultaneously and observed. Parallel studies are used with common disease states where obtaining adequate numbers of participants is not a problem. In addition, parallel group studies are used when treatment effects are anticipated to continue after treatment is discontinued, thus eliminating a crossover design as a possible option (see **Figure 2.1**). Crossover studies are often used to reduce the number of subjects needed to meet statistical power because subjects serve as their own control. In a crossover design, subjects receive a particular treatment for a period of time and then are switched to the alternate treatment. Crossover stud-

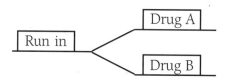

Figure 2.1: Parallel Group Study Design

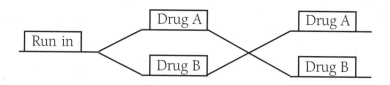

Figure 2.2: Crossover Study Design

ies must allow ample time for washout of the previous treatment to ensure that treatment effects will not be carried over. The effects of each treatment are observed.

A crossover design can greatly reduce inter-subject variability; therefore, the magnitude of effect can be more accurately calculated in this type of study (see **Figure 2.2**). While the crossover design has advantages, it is not appropriate in all disease states. For instance, when mortality is the endpoint for a study, a crossover design where patients are exposed to multiple treatments would confound the results. In fact, patients may die before the crossover period and receive only one treatment. This defeats the purpose of the design.

Another type of crossover trial known as a N of 1 trial involves a single patient or small numbers of patients serving as their own control who receive alternating courses of treatment over a specific period of time. Because such a design involves very small numbers of patients, these studies are limited by generalizability but may be useful in rare disease states or situations in which funding is limited. Although these studies may contain costs, this design often requires an increase in study period to achieve the desired amount of treatment exposure in the subjects. The study period is frequently doubled to allow the subjects to serve as their own control. Caution should be used when applying these results to the general population because the number of patients exposed with this type of design is extremely limited.

Observational Trial Design (Epidemiological Design)

In observational trials, subjects are not assigned an intervention; investigators merely observe subjects and gather information. Subjects are chosen based on presence or absence of specific characteristics. It is extremely difficult to control for confounding variables in these studies. For this reason, cause and effect is difficult to prove and temporal relationships are not easy to establish; therefore, only associations can be observed. Results from observational trials are less reliable than results from interventional trials, but often times will lead to larger interventional studies to examine effects closer in a better controlled environment. **Figure 2.3** shows a diagram of the various observational study designs.

Prospective

In a prospective observational trial design, investigators define the disease and the predicted variables prior to the onset of disease. Subjects are chosen based on specific characteristics, such as smoking, and followed forward in time to observe the development of a specific outcome such as lung cancer. If subjects are followed forward in time, or prospectively, the groups are often referred to as cohorts. One of the largest and well known cohort studies is the Framingham Heart Study. These studies can also be referred to as followup studies, meaning that they begin with a cohort or group and follow the subjects forward in time until the characteristic or disease is observed.

Retrospective

In retrospective observational trial design, investigators define the disease and the predicted variables after disease onset. Retrospective cohort, also known as a trohoc study, examines existing data and looks back in time to determine various characteristics that may have led to disease development. For instance, investigators examine the data for a group of subjects with a diagnosis

Prospective Observational Trials

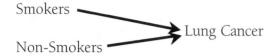

Retrospective Observational Trials

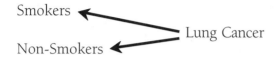

Case Control Studies

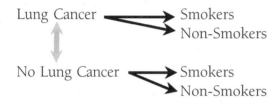

Figure 2.3: Observational Study Designs

of lung cancer and analyze their smoking history to determine if an association exists between smoking and development of lung cancer.

Case Control

In a case control study, investigators look back in time and compare two groups: the cases and controls. Cases are the group that have a specific characteristic or disease, and the controls are chosen as comparison and do not have the characteristic or disease. The investigators aim to determine if there are any characteristics that differ between the two groups such as a history of smoking. In such a study, information can be gathered in various ways, including survey, chart review, and direct interview. Case control studies are useful to gather information regarding rare disorders or disorders in which there is a long period between exposure and development of outcome. Case control studies are especially susceptible to bias, especially if investigators rely on the recall of subjects.

Results of Observational Trials

Results of observational trials are reported by measures of association such as odds or risk ratios, all of which need to be interpreted with caution and a good understanding of the definitions. Risk ratios are calculated on data from prospective trials to determine the risk of an outcome or adverse event in one group compared to another group. Relative risk, relative risk reduction, and absolute risk reduction are all types of risk ratios that need to be interpreted with caution and a good understanding of the definitions.

Relative risk is the risk of an outcome in one group compared to another (see **Figure 2.4**). Relative risk reduction, on the other hand, represents the relative change from baseline in outcome or adverse event rate between intervention and control group (see **Figure 2.5**). Relative risk reduction may elevate the benefit of a treatment because it does not account for the variability of baseline risk between subjects and assumes similar risks for all. Absolute risk reduction is a better representation of the magnitude of effect for a treatment because it takes into account the baseline risks for individual subjects and represents the difference in adverse events between intervention and control groups (see **Figure 2.6**).

$$\text{Relative Risk} = \frac{\text{Outcome or Adverse Event (treatment group)}}{\text{Outcome or Adverse Event (control group)}}$$

Figure 2.4: Relative Risk

$$\text{Relative Risk Reduction} = (1 - \text{Relative Risk})$$

Figure 2.5: Relative Risk Reduction

$$\text{Absolute Risk Reduction} = (\text{Risk in Control Group}) - (\text{Risk in Treatment Group})$$

Figure 2.6: Absolute Risk Reduction

Ultimately, what do all the numbers mean and how do the results apply to patients? Number needed to treat provides a clear illustration of the magnitude of benefit of a specific treatment by providing the number of patients required to prevent one outcome or adverse event (see **Figure 2.7**).

$$\textbf{Number Needed to Treat (NNT)} = \frac{1}{\textbf{Absolute Risk Reduction}}$$

Figure 2.7: Number Needed to Treat

Example 2.1 illustrates how different the numbers can appear.

Example 2.1. Interpreting Risk

A study was designed to compare simvastatin (n=2221) versus placebo (n=2223) and incidence of death from cardiovascular causes. The incidence of death in the simvastatin group was n=182 and placebo n=256.

- Relative Risk = death in simvastatin group ÷ death in placebo group = 182 ÷ 256 = 0.71 (71%)
- Relative Risk Reduction = 1 − RR = 1 − 0.71 = 0.29 (29%)
- Absolute Risk Reduction = risk in placebo group − risk in simvastatin group = 256/2223 − 182/2221 = 0.033 (3.3%)
- Number Needed to Treat = 1 ÷ ARR = 1 ÷ 0.033 = 30

Key Concepts of Trial Design

❑ Controls
  - Placebo control − Placebo control trials demonstrate if a treatment works, but do not establish superiority

over alternative treatments. Placebo controls can be unethical, especially in patients with an established disease such as diabetes. In such a case, an active control would be more appropriate.

- Active control – Active control trials demonstrate if a treatment works and also aid in determining superiority of certain treatments. Often times the "gold standard" therapy is used as the control.

- Historical controls – Historical controls are used when new therapies have been proven better and it is determined that it would be unethical to use a previous treatment as an active control. For instance, it has been determined that an Alzheimer's Disease drug has an effect in reversing the disease. From this, the extent of the effect needs to be determined, but current treatments cannot be used because none of them actually reverse the disease.

❑ Blinding – Appropriate blinding techniques are important to reduce bias; double-blind designs are ideal to ensure that neither the subject nor the investigator is affected by the knowledge of the treatment received. Because it may be impossible to blind treatment in certain situations, steps should be taken to ensure bias does not affect the results of the trial. It is important to be aware of the impact that blinding has and evaluate the results of the trial for bias.

❑ Randomization – Randomization attempts to ensure similar demographics and baseline characteristics and allows confounding variables to be equal between treatment groups.

❑ Inclusion/exclusion criteria

- Appropriate inclusion criteria ensure subjects are included for the target disease state and/or characteristics for which the treatment is intended.

- Appropriate exclusion criteria are important to ensure the safety of subjects in the study.

❑ Outcomes – Appropriate outcome measurements are crucial to applicability of the results of the trial; if outcome
measurements are not appropriate, it is difficult to apply
results of the trial to patient decisions.

Essential Biostatistic Concepts

Statistical Significance

In clinical trial design, a medical intervention and its effects are
usually compared to a different intervention, either a placebo or
an active comparator. In both cases, statistical differences could
exist between groups (e.g., demographic characteristics of the
study groups, therapeutic clinical outcomes, adverse event rates).
When these differences are statistically significant, the likelihood
of them existing due to chance is small.

Note that a calculated statistically significant difference is not
necessarily a clinically important difference between study groups.
For instance, a statistically significant difference may be shown
between study groups with diastolic blood pressures of 78 mmHg
and 81 mmHg; however, this would not necessarily be considered a clinically important difference.

Alpha value

The alpha (α) value is the threshold that, when crossed, indicates a statistically significant difference between treatment groups
is reached. This level of significance is established by the study
investigators prior to the conduct of the study. The arbitrary α
value is commonly set at 5% (0.05). When the value is set higher,
such as 10% (0.10), it could be interpreted as a less rigorous
statistical analysis since the results would be presented in a more
favorable way. If the investigators set the value at 1% (0.01), the
statistical analysis would be interpreted as being more rigorous.

P-value

The p-value is an indicator to demonstrate statistically significant differences between two treatment groups. The **p**-value represents the **p**robability that the statistical difference measured

between treatment groups occurred by chance alone and not the intervention being studied. For instance, a p-value of 0.05 means there is a 5% chance that a difference seen between treatment groups occurred by chance alone. Explained another way, it means there is a 95% chance that the measured difference observed between study groups is real and not due to chance. Statistical tests can be used to determine a calculated p-value, and they are discussed later in this chapter.

Once alpha is set, a p-value that is determined from the statistical test applied to the data is generated and then compared to the alpha value. If the p-value is less than the α level (e.g., p-value < 0.05), the probability of the statistical difference being attributed to random chance is very low (<5%). It indicates a high likelihood that the intervention under study produced a difference in the measure of interest (see **Example 2.2**).

Example 2.2. Determining Statistical Significance

A study was designed to show that a new drug was indeed more effective than the drug considered standard of care for a particular disease state. The investigators set alpha at 0.05. This indicates that the investigators are willing to accept a 5% chance that if a statistically significant difference is noted from this trial, that difference actually may not really exist (Type I error). This is also referred to as a false positive.

The correct statistical test was applied for the type of data represented. The new drug showed an improvement over the standard drug of 37% for the primary outcome measurement. The statistical test generated a p-value of 0.0001 (p=0.0001). With the alpha set at 0.05, this p-value is clearly less than the alpha level and, therefore, the difference noted is statistically significant.

Additional information providing important points to remember regarding p-values and statistical significance can be found at the end of this chapter.

Power

Power is the ability of a study to accurately detect actual differences between treatment groups, when such a difference truly does exist. The higher the power is set for a study, the greater the chance the study will show a difference between groups, if one really exists. The lower the power is set, the greater the chance the study will not show a difference between groups when one actually exists.

It is also important to determine whether or not a per protocol or intent-to-treat analysis was completed when determining whether power is met. A per protocol analysis requires knowing the number of patients that completed the study. An intent-to-treat analysis requires knowing the number of patients randomized into the study groups. Note that a modified intent-to-treat analysis includes specific criteria that must be met once a patient is randomized into the study (e.g., must have received at least one dose of the study drug or had at least one follow-up visit: see **Example 2.3**).

Additional information regarding the components that go into calculating power can be found at the end of this chapter.

Example 2.3. Power Is Met and No Difference Exists

A study was designed and conducted that showed no statistically significant difference in the primary outcome measurement between the two treatment groups (p=0.70; alpha 0.05). Power was set at 80% by the investigators during design of the trial. To meet that power, 250 patients in each group were required. When the study was completed, there were 278 and 267 patients in each treatment group, respectively. The investigators used a per protocol analysis meaning they evaluated the outcome measurement only in those patients completing the duration of the study as indicated in the protocol. Based on this information, power was met so there is an 80% chance that if a difference did exist, this trial would have shown that difference.

If the investigators had set a power of 95% during the design of the trial, this would have required a sample size of 300 patients per group. Note that if the investigators would have completed the study with patient numbers of 300 or greater per group, power would have been met. This situation would have provided the investigators with a 95% chance of the study showing a difference between groups, if one truly existed.

The higher the power is set, the greater confidence exists that the study will be able to correctly detect a difference between groups, if one truly exists. In other words, a power of 95% that is met gives the investigators a greater chance than the 80% power to identify a difference, if one truly exists.

Sample size is the primary factor that an investigator can directly control to achieve a study's set power (see table in **Figure 2.8**). Ironically, sample size is also the primary driver behind the cost and time required to conduct a clinical study. This can often contribute to the reason why many clinical trials do not meet their required power. Enough time and/or money could not be invested to assure a large enough sample size to meet the set power.

The ideal situation is when the investigators set power, and the sample size per group is adequately enrolled/completed to meet that set power. In this case, whether there is a statistically significant difference between treatment groups or not, there *is* confidence that a difference would have been identified if one actually existed (see **Example 2.4**).

Situation	Sample Size Needed to Meet Power	Power Met/ Not Met	Conclusion
Power is set (≥80%).	Identified in article and sample size adequate to meet power.	Met	80% chance that a statistically significant difference between groups will be noted, if one truly exists. Acceptable.
Power is set (≥80%).	Identified in article but sample size not adequate to meet power.	Not Met	<80% chance that a statistically significant difference between groups will be noted, if one truly exists. Not acceptable.
Power is set (≥80%).	Not identified in article.	Not Met (assumption that must be made)	No easy way to verify if sample size was adequate to meet power and detect a statistically significant difference, if one truly exists.
Power mentioned but without details (no mention of %).	Identified in article, but unable to determine if sample size adequate to meet power since actual percentage not revealed.	Not Met (assumption that must be made)	No easy way to verify if power was appropriate (≥80%).
Power is not reported (no mention of %).	Not identified in article and unable to determine if adequate to meet power since power not set.	Not Met (assumption that must be made)	No easy way to verify if sample size was adequate or power was appropriate (≥80%).
Power is claimed to be met, but not reported (no mention of %).	Not identified in article and unable to determine if adequate to meet power since no mention of actual %.	Not Met (assumption that must be made)	No easy way to verify if sample size was adequate or power was appropriate (≥80%).

Figure 2.8: Various Ways that Power and Sample Size Can Be Reported

Example 2.4. Power Is Met and No Difference Exists

A study was designed and conducted that showed no statistically significant difference in the primary outcome measurement between the two treatment groups (p=0.85; alpha 0.05). Power was set at 80% by the investigators during design of the trial. To meet that power, 250 patients in each group were required. There were 270 patients randomized into each treatment group, respectively. The investigators used an intent-to-treat analysis meaning they evaluated the outcome measurement in all those patients randomized into the study. Based on this information, power was met and, therefore, we have an 80% chance of observing a difference between treatment groups, if one really did exist.

Note that if a difference would have been shown in the above study, knowing if power was met is not as crucial since enough patients completed the trial to actually show a difference.

If the results of a study conclude that no statistically significant differences exist between treatment groups, then it is imperative to verify that power was set and met. The validity of the study's results becomes questionable if power was set but not met with the necessary number of patients enrolled/completed in the trial. In the following example (see **Example 2.5**), the study did not have a large enough sample size to meet power and therefore, detect actual differences if they really existed. When this happens, inaccurate conclusions can be made by the investigators that no difference exists when one really may exist.

Example 2.5. Power Not Met and No Difference Exists

A study was designed and conducted that showed no statistically significant difference in the primary outcome measurement between the two treatment groups (p=0.16; alpha 0.05). Power was set at 80% by the investigators during design of the trial. To meet that power, 250 patients in each group were required. When the study was completed, there were 207 and 228 patients in each treatment group, respectively. The investigators used a per protocol analysis meaning they evaluated the outcome measurement only in those patients completing the duration of the study as indicated in the protocol. Based on this information, power was not met and we cannot be sure that a difference may exist if enough patients would have been entered into the study to meet power.

If the results concluded that a statistically significant difference did exist between treatment groups, power becomes less of a concern because power is associated with an actual difference being detected if one exists (see **Example 2.6**). The important question in this situation is whether the study participants' characteristics are representative of the larger target population planned for the treatment being tested. Clinical judgment is required to make the correct decision in this situation.

Example 2.6. Power Not Met and Difference Exists

A study was designed and conducted that showed a statistically significant difference in the primary outcome measurement between the two treatment groups (p=0.0012; alpha 0.05). Power was set at 80% by the investigators during design of the trial.

To meet that power, 250 patients in each group were required. When the study was completed, there were 233 and 241 patients in each treatment group, respectively. The investigators used a per protocol analysis meaning they evaluated the outcome measurement only in those patients completing the duration of the study as indicated in the protocol. Based on this information, power was not met. However, enough patients were evidently entered into the trial to show a statistically significant difference so not meeting the set power is less of a concern.

Figure 2.9 illustrates various power scenarios that can occur when a statistically significant difference between groups does or does not exist. In addition, the reliability of the study results in each of these scenarios is provided.

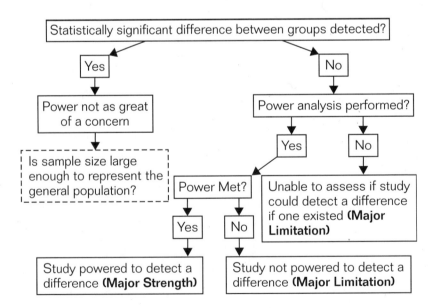

Figure 2.9: Power Scenarios

Appropriate Test for Data Analyzed

A study must use the appropriate statistical test for the type of data being analyzed to assure the integrity of the results. To fully understand this concept, a basic knowledge of data types and data distribution is required.

Types of data

Data or variable scales consist of four different types of measurement: interval, ratio, ordinal, and nominal. **Figure 2.10** provides a definition summary table of each type of data and respective data distribution.

Interval and ratio data are both considered "continuous" data scales, having a known, equal distance between each data point. Interval data scales can contain negative numbers. An example includes temperature measured in the Celsius or Fahrenheit scale. Ratio data scales contain no negative numbers. Examples of ratio data include age, weight, serum glucose, blood pressure, and incidence rates of outcomes. Ratio data can also be described in "ratios" since there are no negative numbers. Even though technical differences exist, it is important to know that interval and ratio data are handled the same way when selecting the most appropriate statistical tests.

Ordinal data are data that can be ranked in a specific order. This type of data differs from continuous data because the distance between data points are not equal. An example of ordinal data is a Likert-type scale, where a patient's mood is measured in ranked order as no agitation, mild agitation, moderate agitation, or extreme agitation.

Nominal data are also categorical data, but cannot be ranked like ordinal data. Two subgroups of nominal data are binomial and non-binomial. Nominal data that has only two possible outcomes is called "binomial" data. For instance, binomial nominal data is commonly used when measuring mortality and full recovery (either it happened or it did not). Non-binomial nominal data has more than two possible outcomes, but still cannot be ranked like ordinal data. For instance, non-binomial nominal data includes eye color (blue, brown, hazel) and various ethnicities.

Type of Data	Definition	Examples	Data Distribution	Type of Statistical Test Used
Interval	Continuous data scales with known, equal distance between each interval; they can contain negative numbers.	Temperature (Fahrenheit and Celcius)	Usually normal distribution (also known as parametric distribution).	Parametric unless the data is skewed; then non-parametric may be appropriate.
Ratio	Continuous data scales with known, equal distance between each interval; they contain a non-arbitrary, absolute zero (i.e., no negative numbers).	Age, weight, serum glucose, blood pressure, and incidence rates of outcomes	Usually normal distribution (also known as parametric distribution).	Parametric unless the data is skewed; then non-parametric may be appropriate.
Ordinal	Data that can be ranked in specific order. The intervals between data points are not equal distance.	Likert-type pain scale where pain is ranked as no pain, moderate pain, and extreme pain	Non-normal distribution (also known as non-parametric distribution).	Non-parametric
Nominal	Categorical data that cannot be ranked. "Binomial" nominal data has only two outcomes.	Eye color, ethnicity, and gender Mortality and full recovery (either happened or did not)	Both nominal and binomial nominal data have non-normal distribution (also known as non-parametric distribution).	Non-parametric for both nominal and binomial nominal.

Figure 2.10: Types of Data to Be Analyzed

Each type of data represents a specific distribution when plotted on a graph. See **Figure 2.11** for a visual example of each type of distribution. The two most important types of distribution are parametric (normal) distribution and non-parametric (non-normal) distribution (see **Example 2.7**).

> ## Example 2.7. Normal and Non-Normal Data Distribution
>
> An example of normal distribution would be to plot the height of the students in a typical pharmacy school class. If this sample of students had evenly distributed characteristics, this plot could represent the normal distribution of heights for the entire college campus.
>
> This same example can serve to illustrate a non-normal distribution. This situation would be to plot the height of the students in that same pharmacy school class in addition to including the basketball team. When looking at this distribution of heights, one can see that the height is not normally distributed. The addition of several of the tallest students on the college campus has skewed the distribution. The addition of a group not representative of the overall college campus confounds the normal distribution and distributes the height data in a non-normal manner.

Statistical tests applied to data

Statistical tests applied to data are described as being either parametric or non-parametric in nature. In general, continuous data (interval and ratio) should be analyzed using parametric statistical tests, and categorical data (ordinal and nominal) should be analyzed using non-parametric statistical tests. Each type of statistical test has an underlying set of assumptions to the data being analyzed. Parametric tests assume a normal distribution, while non-parametric tests do not make assumptions about the distri-

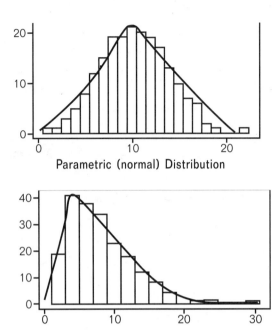

Parametric (normal) Distribution

Positive Non-parametric (non-normal) Distribution

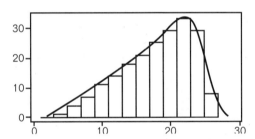

Negative Non-parametric (non-normal) Distribution

Figure 2.11: Parametric and Non-Parametric Data Distributions

bution of data. As long as these assumptions are met, then the statistical tests can provide accurate results (see **Figure 2.12**).

If an investigator uses a parametric statistical test for categorical data, the results of that statistical test are questionable and one must assess them cautiously in making any conclusive statements. Technically, it is inappropriate to use parametric statistical tests on categorical data. Parametric tests have an underlying assumption of normal distribution using continuous data. Categorical data have a non-normal distribution and, therefore, do not fit the underlying assumption for the parametric test.

In special situations, non-parametric tests may be used to analyze continuous data such as when data has become non-normally distributed or "skewed." When this is noted, it should be questioned why the investigators would use a non-parametric test to analyze normally distributed continuous data.

In general, parametric statistical tests should be used for continuous data that is normally distributed (interval and ratio data). Non-parametric statistical tests are used for types of data where no assumption of normal distribution can or is being made.

The table in **Figure 2.13** assists the practitioner in determining which common statistical tests may be used for interval, ratio, ordinal, and nominal data. If a statistical test is not listed in the table, one should refer to other statistical resources listed as references for this chapter. In the event that this strategy fails, a quick search on the Internet using the statistical test in question as the search term can also be useful.

The following **Examples 2.8–2.10** provide an opportunity to utilize the table found in Figure 2.13 and become familiar with the above concepts of parametric and non-parametric data and tests.

Example 2.8. Appropriate Test for Type of Data Analyzed

In a particular trial, patients were randomly assigned to one of two groups: Drug A or Drug B group, respectively. To measure the effect that each drug had on controlling blood glucose levels after a meal, serum glucose levels were drawn at set times after the meal. These serum glucose levels were the primary outcome measure for this study. The statistical methodology section stated that a Student's t-test was used to determine if a statistically significant difference was seen between Drug A and Drug B in the reduction of serum glucose levels after the 3-month trial.

In this example, serum glucose levels are the data being collected as the primary outcome.

Type of Data: (serum glucose levels) Continuous data having a known, equal distance between each interval and containing a non-arbitrary, absolute zero (i.e., no negative numbers). This is considered **ratio data**.

Appropriate Test: (Student's t-test) Yes, according to the table in Figure 2.13; Student's t-test (a parametric test) can be used with ratio data (normal distribution).

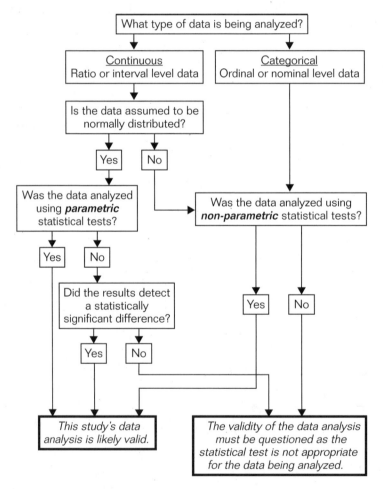

Figure 2.12: Statistical Test Decision Flowchart

Nominal	Ordinal	Continuous (Ratio or Interval)
• Chi-Square test (x^2) • Cochran's Q test • Fischer's exact test • Logistic Regression • Mantel-Haenszel • McNemar's test	• ANCOVA ranks • ANOVA ranks • Friedman ANOVA • Kendal Rank correlation coefficient • Kruskal-Wallis ANOVA • Mann-Whitney U test • Spearman Rank correlation coefficient • Wilcoxin Rank Sum test • Wilcoxin Signed Rank test	• ANCOVA • ANOVA • Pearson Correlation Coefficient (r) • Student's t-test

Figure 2.13: Commonly Used Parametric and Non-Parametric Statistical Tests by Type of Data Analyzed *Note that each of these tests has its own underlying assumptions and are sometimes meant for very specific situations, depending upon the study design and type of data being analyzed. Please refer to statistical textbook references to learn more about these specific tests and when they are appropriately applied.*

Example 2.9. Inappropriate Test for Type of Data Analyzed

A study was conducted to measure an investigational drug's effect on decreasing agitation in bipolar children. The comparison group was standard therapy. Each child's caregiver was asked to rate the amount of agitation at set times over the 8-week trial as no agitation, mild agitation, moderate agitation, or severe agitation. The statistical test used to determine if there was a statistically significant difference between the two drugs for reducing agitation was a Chi-square test.

In this example, the primary outcome measure was a Likert scale measuring the degree of agitation.

Type of Data: (Likert scale) Categorical data that can be ranked in a specific order and the intervals between data points are not equal in distance. This is considered ordinal data.

Appropriate Test: (Chi-square test) No, according to the table in Figure 2.13; Chi-square test should be used with nominal data, not ordinal data. Note that a non-parametric test was being used for data that is non-normal in distribution; however, additional assumptions made with this type of test (used with categorical data that cannot be ranked) did not fit the data being analyzed which was categorical and ranked data.

Example 2.10. Inappropriate Test for Type of Data Analyzed

In a trial designed to show if the standard of therapy prevented the incidence of myocardial infarctions, hospitalizations, and/or death, patients on this standard of therapy were followed over a 3-year period after angioplasty and stent placement. Patient or patient's family member completed a questionnaire provided monthly asking if the patient experienced a myocardial infarction or hospitalization due to a cardiovascular event. In addition, caregivers were asked in this questionnaire if the patient was still alive or not. The statistical section stated that a two-way analysis of variance (ANOVA) was used to analyze these primary outcome measures.

The primary outcome measures were whether a patient experienced a myocardial infarction, hospitalization, and/or death.

Type of Data: (occurred or didn't occur) Categorical data that cannot be ranked and has only two outcomes (either it happened or it did not). This is binomial nominal data.

Appropriate Test: (Two-way ANOVA) No, according to the table in Figure 2.13; this test (parametric test) is not used with nominal (non-parametric) data.

Key Idea

In general, parametric statistical tests should be used for continuous data (interval and ratio data) that is normally distributed. Non-parametric statistical tests can be used for other types of data where no assumption of normal distribution can or is being made.

Summary

This chapter describes practical applications of basic concepts required for interpretation of clinical research results. Various study designs are used in clinical research. Understanding the type of study design described in an article allows identification of strengths and weaknesses within the design that could affect accurate interpretation of the results.

Correct interpretation of biostatistics applied to the results of a study can sometimes be difficult. Knowing the relationship between alpha and p-values allows confirmation of claims being made by the investigators. In addition, knowing that a study is adequately powered provides confidence in results showing no difference between treatment groups. Finally, being able to determine if the appropriate statistical test is used for the type of data being analyzed gives assurance that reported statistically significant differences really do exist between treatment groups.

Understanding these concepts is required to work the 5-Step

Evidence-Based Medicine Process described in this book. Without a working knowledge of these essential concepts in study design and biostatistics, practitioners could inaccurately interpret trial results that may lead to inappropriate and potentially unsafe clinical decisions.

References

1. Norman GR, Streiner DL. *PDQ Statistics*. 3rd ed. Hamilton, London (Ontario): BC Decker Inc.; 2003.

2. Elenbass RM, Elenbass JK, Cuddy PG. Evaluating the medical literature. Part 2: Statistical analysis. *Ann Emerg Med*. 1983; 12(10):610–620.

3. Gaddis ML, Gaddis GM. Introduction to biostatistics: Part 1, basic concepts. *Ann Emerg Med*. 1990; 19:86–89.

4. Gaddis GM, Gaddis ML. Introduction to biostatistics: Part 2, descriptive statistics. *Ann Emerg Med*. 1990; 19:309–315.

5. Gaddis GM, Gaddis ML. Introduction to biostatistics: Part 3, sensitivity, specificity, predictive value and hypothesis testing. *Ann Emerg Med*. 1990; 19:591–597.

6. Gaddis GM, Gaddis ML. Introduction to biostatistics: Part 4, statistical inference techniques in hypothesis testing. *Ann Emerg Med*. 1990; 19:820–825.

7. Gaddis GM, Gaddis ML. Introduction to biostatistics: Part 5, statistical inference techniques for hypothesis testing with non parametric data. *Ann Emerg Med*. 1990; 19:1054–1059.

8. Gaddis ML, Gaddis GM. Introduction to biostatistics: Part 6, correlation and regression. *Ann Emerg Med*. 1990; 19:1462–1468.

9. Riegelman RK. *Studying a Study and Testing a Test*. 4th ed. Philadelphia, PA: Lippincott Williams & Wilkins; 2000.

10. Gehlbach SH. *Interpreting the Medical Literature*. 4th ed. New York, NY: McGraw-Hill; 2002.

11. Friedman LM, Furberg CD, DeMets DL. *Fundamentals of Clinical Trial.* 3rd ed. New York, NY: Springer; 1998.

12. Glantz SA. *Primer of Biostatistics.* 6th ed. New York, NY: McGraw-Hill; 2005.

13. Hulley SB, Cummings SR, Browner WS, et al. *Designing Clinical Research.* 3rd ed. Philadelphia, PA: Lippincott Williams and Wilkins; 2007.

Significance and p-Values

The following are important points to remember regarding p-values and statistical significance:

1. P-values cannot be used as absolute proof that an intervention has a particular benefit or not. The only way to fully eliminate random chance as a contributor to study results is to enroll the entire worldly population being studied. Also, unknown confounding variables that have nothing to do with the intervention(s) being studied could have contributed to the measured statistical differences. This is why proper study design to minimize confounding variables is so important.

2. No matter how small the difference, any difference of effect between groups can be considered statistically significant if the study design's power is high enough (see section on Power in this chapter).

3. When attempting to compare various treatments and their associated effects based on clinical trial results, it is *not appropriate* to compare p-values as a way to determine which intervention is safer or more efficacious. P-values do not equate to levels of magnitude.

Components of Power

Power is related to another concept, the Beta (β) Level. The β level is the probability of making a Type II Error, or falsely determining that no actual difference exists between two study groups when a difference truly does exist (i.e., "false negative"). For example, a β level of 20% (or 0.2) means that there is a 20% probability that the study will falsely determine that no difference exists between groups when a difference truly does exist. *How is β related to power?* Conceptually, power can be calculated as $1 - \beta$. Using our previous example of β set at 20%, then the resultant power of the study is calculated as $1 - 0.2$, which equals 0.8 or 80%. A study having an estimated power of 80% means that the study has an 80% chance of seeing a difference between treatment groups, if a difference really exists. **Power set at 80% is considered appropriate for most studies**; however, often 85% to 90% power is set for high investment studies (e.g., long-term, large trials, etc.).

While $1 - \beta$ is a very simplistic way of calculating power, complex equations are used when attempting to quantify the true statistical power of a study based on several factors. Components that go into a power calculation include:

- ❏ Level of significance (α) – *usually set at 0.05*
- ❏ Type II Error Rate (β) – *usually set at 0.20*
- ❏ Magnitude of difference in an outcome measure between treatment groups (δ) – *usually obtained from previous studies using the intervention if it exists; if not, then much more speculative*
- ❏ Variability (σ)
- ❏ Sample size (n)

These are the primary components of a power calculation. There are several other components that may be considered by experienced biostatisticians that involve far more complex concepts than what is covered within the scope of this book.

Define

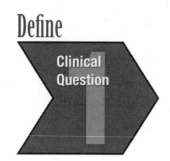

Clinical
Question

Chapter 3

Define the Clinical Question

Patrick J. Bryant

Step 1 – Define the Clinical Question

The first step of the 5-Step Evidence-Based Medicine Process, Define the Clinical Question, may be the most difficult one because it involves the translation of a clinical problem into an answerable clinical question. Defining and structuring an appropriate clinical question are both critical. According to a survey conducted by the Drug Information Service at the Medical College of Virginia Hospitals, the original clinical question asked was significantly different from the actual question that needed to be answered 85% of the time.[1] This problem suggests the need for applying some type of systematic process to ensure the most accurate definition of the clinical question. One approach using a logical and systematic manner to define the problem and clarify the clinical question has been proposed by drug information specialists.[2] The goal of this approach is to understand the *context* and *scope* of the problem.

85% of the time the original clinical question identified is significantly different from the actual question needing to be answered.

Framing the Clinical Question Using PICO

Accurately defining the clinical question is essential to providing direction for the remaining four steps of the evidence-based medicine process outlined in this book. Those steps include retrieving the pertinent literature, critically evaluating the literature, categorizing the quality of the evidence, and developing a recommendation that can be justified. A generic, minimally defined clinical question does not provide the required direction for these steps.

Example 3.1. Using Minimal Detail to Define the Clinical Questions

An example of a generic, minimally detailed clinical question is taking a newly marketed non-injectable insulin product and asking if this product should be added to a preferred drug list within an institution. The following can be determined from this minimal information:

1. **context** – a preferred drug list formulary management activity for an institution

2. **scope** – a population-based decision for a specific institution that may have a particular patient population such as indigent and/or Medicaid

With this example, only the context and scope of the question are provided. The details necessary to define the true clinical question are missing. Using the PICO approach, the definitive details of the clinical question can be determined.

An accepted approach for framing the clinical question is provided by Sackett and colleagues using an acronym approach referred to as PICO.[3-5] This approach includes the following components:

Patients – What individual patient or patient population is associated with the clinical question? Are there any patient subgroups that require special attention?

Interventions – What interventions can be used in this clinical situation?

Comparison – What additional interventions can be considered and compared to the chosen intervention?

Outcome – What is the end result most desired for the individual patient, patient population, and/or patient subgroup?

The specific patient group, therapeutic options to consider, and desired results of using a specific therapeutic option must be identified when defining the clinical question. **Figure 3.1** (see also the "EBM Tool Kit" at the end of this book) details the PICO process and the resulting benefits of using this approach.

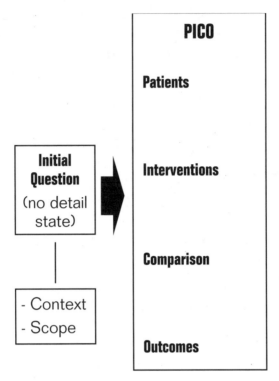

Figure 3.1: PICO Illustration

Example 3.2. PICO Approach Defined

The Patient population includes both type 1 and 2 diabetics either just initiating therapy or having been on insulin for a period of time. A special subgroup of patients to consider might include those with a "needle phobia" or those who want a more practical way to administer insulin when out in public.

The Intervention is the non-injectable insulin. Related questions would further define how the intervention is administered and provide a description of the device needed for administration, frequency of administration, and dosing equivalency to injectable insulin.

The Comparison includes injectable insulins and other interventions such as competitor non-injectable insulins, insulin stimulators, and insulin enhancers. Also a review of alternatives to the non-injectable insulin represented by the Intervention is performed.

The Outcome is adequate glycemic control as measured by fasting blood glucose levels and HbA_{1C} without the problems and inconveniences associated with injectable insulin (See **Figure 3.2**).

Using this PICO approach now allows development of a well-defined clinical question as illustrated in **Example 3.3**.

Example 3.3: The Well-Defined Clinical Question

"Are there safety and/or convenience benefits associated with this non-injectable insulin compared to injectable insulin, other non-injectable insulins, insulin stimulators, or insulin enhancers to provide normal blood glucose and glycemic control in type 1 and 2 diabetic patients? Is there a difference in patient motivation to use the non-injectable insulin between patients just initiating versus maintaining insulin therapy and/or those patients with 'needle phobia'?"

Effects on Other Evidence-Based Medicine Activities

Once the clinical question has been accurately defined, the following activities associated with the evidence-based medicine process can be initiated.

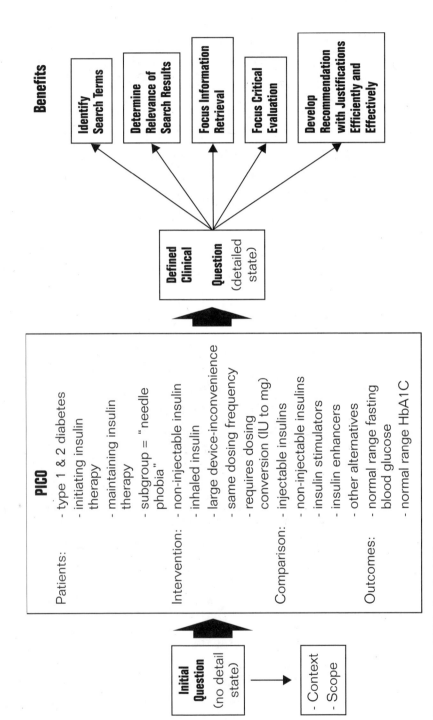

Figure 3.2: PICO Applied Illustration

❑ Identify specific search terms for use in retrieving pertinent information (see **Example 3.4**).

Example 3.4. Specific Search Terms

- The specific intervention's trade name
- Names of other competing non-injectable insulins
- Names of insulin stimulators
- Names of insulin enhancers
- Names of injectable insulins
- Type 1 diabetes
- Type 2 diabetes
- Fasting blood glucose
- HbA_{1C}
- "Needle phobia"

❑ Determine the relevance of the search results now that the details of the patient population, intervention, comparisons, and desired outcomes are known.

❑ Focus information retrieval and critical evaluation efforts toward the pertinent evidence as the specific patient population, intervention, comparison, and desired outcomes have been identified by the defined clinical question.

❑ Develop a recommendation more efficiently and effectively based on observations made possible by a well-defined clinical question during the critical evaluation of the evidence (see **Example 3.5**).

Example 3.5. Specific Observations

- Determine if there are safety and/or convenience benefits associated with using non-injectable insulin versus identified alternative therapies.

- Determine if there is a difference in patient motivation to use a non-injectable insulin between type 1 and type 2 diabetic patients.

- Determine if there is a difference in patient motivation to use a non-injectable insulin in patients initiating injectable insulin therapy for the first time versus patients already maintained on injectable insulin.

- Consider if a subgroup of patients with "needle phobia" is more likely to utilize the non-injectable insulin compared to those without this problem.

Key Idea

A well-defined clinical question assists in identifying search terms, determining relevance of the search results, performing a critical evaluation of the evidence, and developing a recommendation.

Tips for Defining the Clinical Question

Important points to consider when defining the clinical question include the following:

❑ Describe a group of patients with similar characteristics as those in the problem or situation you are trying to define with the clinical question.

❑ Identify the primary intervention.

❑ Identify the most likely alternative intervention(s) to be considered.

❑ Identify the primary desired outcome and how that outcome is measured in the clinical setting.

Problems to Be Avoided

Finally, some common problems are associated with defining the clinical question that should be avoided:

❑ Complex clinical situations resulting in numerous questions identified can be handled by dissecting the situation into smaller, less complex, and more manageable problems requiring fewer questions.

❑ Too little or complete lack of adequate background information can be handled by further questioning key people associated with the clinical situation.

❑ Lack of time to complete an evidence-based medicine analysis can be due to an overabundance of clinical problems associated with the situation. Judicious prioritization identifying those clinical problems having the greatest impact on a patient or institution is one way to deal with this issue.

Summary

Defining the clinical question must be done accurately. In addition, this step must be completed with enough detail to provide the required information necessary to conduct the other four steps of the evidence-based medicine process described in this book. An acronym-based approach, referred to as PICO, can be used to assist in defining the clinical question. The PICO approach provides a well-defined clinical question. This clinical question assists in identifying search terms for retrieval of pertinent information and in determining relevance of search results. In addition, focusing information retrieval, focusing critical evaluation efforts, and maximizing efficiency and effectiveness of recommendation development is accomplished with a well-defined clinical question. Clearly, defining the clinical question accurately is the foundation to the entire evidence-based medicine process.

References

1. Kirkwood CF, Kier KL. Modified Systematic Approach to Answering Questions. In: Malone PM, Kier KL, Stanovich JE, eds. *Drug Information: A Guide for Pharmacists*. 3rd ed. New York, NY: McGraw-Hill Companies, Inc; 2006.

2. Calis KA, Sheehan AH. Formulating Effective Responses and Recommendations: A Structured Approach. In: Malone PM, Kier KL, Stanovich JE, eds. *Drug Information: A Guide for Pharmacists*. 3rd ed. New York, NY: McGraw-Hill Companies, Inc; 2006.

3. Sackett DL, Richardson WS, Rosenberg WMC, et al. *Evidence-based Medicine: How to Practice and Teach EBM*. 2nd ed. London: Churchill-Livingstone; 2000.

4. Richardson WS, Wilson MC, Nishikawa J, et al. The well-built clinical question: a key to evidence-based decisions. *ACP J Club*. 1995; 123:A12–A13.

5. Oxman AD, Sackett DL, Guyatt GH. Users' guide to the medical literature. *JAMA*. 1993; 270:2093–2097.

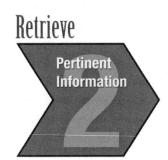

Retrieve

Pertinent
Information

Chapter 4

Retrieve Pertinent Information

**Heather A. Pace, Lindsey N. Schnabel,
Morgan L. Sperry, & Patrick J. Bryant**

Step 2 – Retrieve Pertinent Information

The second step of this 5-Step Evidence-Based Medicine Process, Retrieving Pertinent Information, involves creating a comprehensive search strategy to identify all of the pertinent evidence available relative to the clinical question. This information can be retrieved from a variety of databases and compendia. To complete this step, the pharmacy practitioner needs a basic understanding of common databases and standard search strategies. An incomplete search strategy may cause the omission of key information and may result in an inappropriate recommendation affecting the treatment and/or safety of the patient. Once this strategy is defined and completed, the next step is to refine the search results. Search strategies and the techniques used to organize search results will be discussed in this chapter. Retrieving Pertinent Information is an extremely important step in the 5-Step Evidence-Based Medicine Process because it builds the foundation for this process.

An incomplete search strategy can result in an inappropriate recommendation directly affecting the patient's care.

Deciding Where to Start

To ensure that recommendations are supported by the best available evidence, it is important for a clinical practitioner to understand the steps used to provide a successful search. An effective search strategy begins broad with the use of tertiary resources and narrows to primary resources. Tertiary resources include textbooks and compendia (e.g., Micromedex, LexiComp, Clinical Pharmacology, Facts and Comparisons). These resources are used for gathering general background information pertaining to the clinical question.

Secondary resources are indexing and abstracting services that simplify the search and identify primary literature. Some examples include PubMed (or Medline), International Pharmaceutical Abstracts, Iowa Drug Information Services, and EMBASE. Primary resources refer to journals containing original research, including randomized controlled trials, review articles, case studies, and meta analyses. The resources discussed above are crucial in carrying out the 5-Step Evidence-Based Medicine Process.

Many references mentioned in this chapter are not available to the clinical practitioner; however, they are often available in drug information centers and health science libraries. For this reason, it is important to develop a relationship with a drug information specialist or medical librarian to ensure a comprehensive and high quality search.

For a general review of resources and searching techniques, the reader is directed to the references in this chapter. These references provide a comprehensive review of medical information sources such as commercially available databases and directions for searching them.

Creating the Search Strategy

Broad to narrow search

A precise search strategy is critical to ensure all pertinent evidence is identified.[17,18] Too much or too little detail in the search strategy can result in limited usable evidence. For instance, specific search terms can limit the results while the use of more general search terms often provides excessive amounts of non-relevant information.

Example 4.1. Using General and Specific Search Terms

The defined clinical question is whether Drug A is as effective as Drug B regarding improvement of bone density in the treatment of osteoporosis.

Specific Search Terms:
Drug A brand name

Drug B brand name

General Search Terms:
Drug A generic name

Drug B generic name

Osteoporosis

Bone Density

Drug A—all approved indications besides osteoporosis

Drug B—all approved indications besides osteoporosis

1. Use of specific search terms listed above can limit the search to those articles where only the brand name appears. More possible "hits"

may appear if the search is made somewhat more general by searching both the brand and generic names of Drug A and Drug B.

2. Searching by brand and generic names of Drug B could result in too general of a search if Drug B has been on the market long enough to lose patent exclusivity. In this case, not all the generic products identified with this search are going to be pertinent to the situation. For instance, if the brand name product is the only oral form and this is the route pertinent to the clinical question, then only the brand name drug would be of interest. This is often the case with standard or accepted treatment.

Bibliographic searching

Once the original search is complete, a technique referred to as bibliographic searching can aid in optimizing results of the search. The technique involves reviewing citations of previously identified pertinent information in the original search. This technique can help identify additional literature as well as help in discovering additional search terms that may be useful to broaden the original search. Bibliographic searching helps create a network or "spider web" of information relating to the subject and helps ensure search results are thorough and complete, thus leading to a strong and confident recommendation.

Key Idea

Bibliographic searching ensures thorough and complete search results.

Organizing Search Results—Search and Sift Technique

Applying the skills in Step 4 – Categorize the Quality of Evidence to the retrieval process can maximize efficiency of the literature search and make an overwhelming list of search results manageable. A technique referred to as "Search and Sift" helps the clinician prioritize and organize search results by the quality of evidence and allows evidence to be eliminated that is not pertinent to the clinical question.

The technique involves "sifting" through the abstracts of search results using key words identified from the Ten Major Considerations to quickly determine the quality of evidence (see Chapter 5: Step 3 – Evaluate Literature). This technique also helps eliminate lower quality, less reliable evidence. It is another way in which the 5-Step Evidence-Based Medicine Process outlined in this book helps optimize the clinical decision making and recommendation process (see **Figure 4.1**).

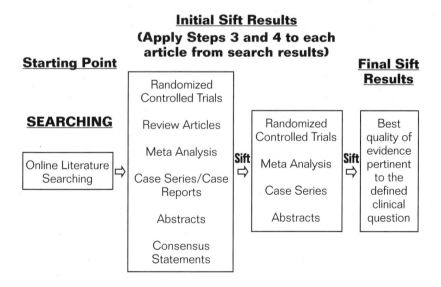

Figure 4.1. "Search and Sift" Strategy

Example 4.2. Using the "Search and Sift" Technique

As a practitioner, you have been asked to provide guidance on the prophylaxis of stress ulcers. After identifying and reviewing the available therapeutic guidelines on stress ulcers, you determine the need to update the original evidence-based guidelines published in 1998. You will need to first retrieve the pertinent information that has become available since this guideline was published.

To help you with this project, you contact a colleague in the drug information center and request a search of the literature for anything that could be used to update this existing 1998 guideline. You receive results of an online literature search. At this point, you also perform a bibliographic search. Because you are proficient using your evidence-based medicine skills, you employ the "Search and Sift" technique and are able to review the abstracts to determine the quality of evidence of the studies and then eliminate evidence that will not help form and support a strong recommendation. You are able to quickly identify six pertinent articles from the 25 results that your colleague identified with the original search (see **Figure 4.2**).

Key Idea

A technique referred to "Search and Sift" helps the clinician prioritize and organize search results by quality of evidence and allows evidence to be eliminated that is not pertinent to the clinical question.

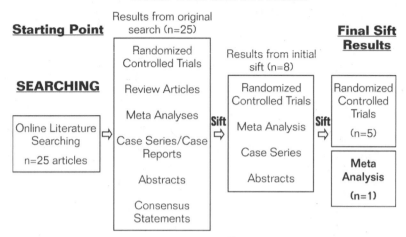

Figure 4.2. "Search and Sift" Strategy for Stress Ulcer Practice Guideline Update

Using the Internet as a Resource

Search results available from various Internet search engines, such as Google, should be used with caution. Because the Internet is so widely available, the source of information is not always clear nor is the information always accurate and/or reliable. A good example is Wikipedia, an online "dictionary" which allows any individual to contribute regardless of the source or validity of information. Additionally, not all medical literature is indexed on the Internet, further limiting the results of the search. In remote cases, a general Internet search may be useful; however, caution is advised. Results from the Internet should be reserved as the last resort only after an exhaustive search of appropriate databases has been completed.

Several factors should be considered before using information obtained from the Internet in an evidence-based medicine analysis[16]:

1. Documented medical evidence is present with citations, not just opinions

2. Website credibility

3. Author's credibility

4. Date of publication

5. Unbiased tone used

6. Peer reviewed

Key Idea

The Internet should be reserved as the last resort only after an exhaustive search of appropriate databases has been completed.

Summary

Retrieving the most pertinent information to be used in the 5-Step Evidence-Based Medicine Process is crucial to making the most accurate recommendation. This is important because these recommendations affect the health and safety of patients. Today's practitioner must rely on drug information specialists and medical librarians to assist with this step. This will ensure the most accurate and comprehensive search results without consuming extensive time from the practitioner. Additional articles found in the reference citations of studies identified by the search can increase the practitioner's confidence that a comprehensive search has been achieved. To optimize efficiency of the search, the practitioner should adopt the "Search and Sift" technique to prioritize and organize search results by quality of evidence. Finally, caution must be used when including information obtained directly from the Internet.

References

1. Shields KM, Lust E. Drug Information Resources. In: Malone PM, Kier KL, Stanovich JE, eds. *Drug Information:*

A Guide for Pharmacists. 3rd ed. New York, NY: McGraw-Hill Companies, Inc; 2006.

2. Malone PM. Electronic Information Management. In: Malone PM, Kier KL, Stanovich JE, eds. *Drug Information: A Guide for Pharmacists.* 3rd ed. New York, NY: McGraw-Hill Companies, Inc; 2006.

3. Greenhalgh T. *How to Read a Paper.* Oxford, UK: Blackwell Publishing Ltd; 2006.

4. Brice A, Palmer J, Bexon N. Information Sourcing. In: Hamer S, Collinson G, eds. *Achieving Evidence-based Practice: A Handbook for Practitioners.* 2nd ed. London, UK: Elsevier Limited; 2005.

5. Chiquette E. Searching the Biomedical Literature: Finding a Needle in a Haystack. In: Chiquette E, Posey LM, eds. *Evidence-Based Pharmacotherapy.* Washington, DC: American Pharmacists Association; 2007.

6. McManus RJ. Sources of Information. In: McGovern DPB, Valori RM, Summerskill WSM, et al., eds. *Key Topics in Evidence-based Medicine.* Oxford, UK: BIOS Scientific Publishers Limited; 2001.

7. Safranek S, Dodson S. Strategies for Finding Evidence. In: Geyman JP, Deyo RA, Ramsey SD, eds. *Evidence-based Clinical Practice: Concepts and Approaches.* Boston, MA: Butterworth Heinemann; 2000.

8. Pirozzo S. Searching the Medical Literature. In: Mayer D, ed. *Essential Evidence-based Medicine.* Cambridge, UK: Cambridge University Press; 2004.

9. Katcher BS. *Medline: A Guide to Effective Searching in PubMed and Other Interfaces.* 2nd ed. San Francisco, CA: Ashbury Press; 2006.

10. Detwiler SM. *Super Searchers on Health & Medicine: The Online Secrets of Top Health & Medical Researchers.* Medford, NJ: Cyberage Books; 2000.

11. Liu JH. Guides to an efficient search for the best evidence. *Seminars in Reproductive Medicine.* 2003; 21(1):5–8.

12. Murphy LS, Reinsch S, Najm WI, et al. Searching biomedical databases on complementary medicine: the use of controlled vocabulary among authors, indexers, and investigators. *BMC Complementary & Alternative Medicine*. 2003; 3:3.

13. Dixon RA, Munro JF, Silcocks PB. *The Evidence Based Medicine Workbook: Critical Appraisal for Clinical Problem Solving*. Oxford, UK: Butterworth – Heinemann; 1997.

14. Glasziou P, Del Mar C, Salisbury J. *Evidence-based Medicine Workbook: Finding and Applying the Best Research Evidence to Improve Patient Care*. London, UK: BMJ Publishing Group; 2003.

15. Guyatt G, Rennie D, eds. *User's Guides to the Medical Literature*. Chicago, IL: AMA Press; 2002.

16. University of Kentucky College of Pharmacy Drug Information. Assessment of quality of internet sites. Available at: www.mc.uky.edu/pharmacy/dic/assessment_sites. html. Accessed October 4, 2007.

17. Heneghan C, Badenoch D. *Evidence-based Medicine Toolkit*. Oxford, UK: Blackwell Publishing Limited; 2006.

18. Levi M. Formulating Clinical Questions. In: McGovern DPB, Summerskill WSM, Valori RM, et al. *Key Topics in Evidence-Based Medicine*. Oxford, UK: BIOS Scientific Publishers Limited; 2001.

19. Pace HA. Evidence-based practice guidelines: Pearls for the clinician. Paper presented at: American Society of Health-System Pharmacists Annual Midyear Clinical Meeting; December 4, 2006; Anaheim, CA.

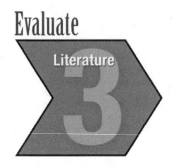

Evaluate

Chapter 5

Evaluate Literature

Morgan L. Sperry & Patrick J. Bryant

Step 3 – Evaluate Literature

After the clinical question has been defined and all pertinent information in answering it has been retrieved, the practitioner will perform a critical literature evaluation on all primary material collected. This third step in the 5-Step Evidence-Based Medicine Process is vital to determine any major limitations in a study and the impact they may have on the results and/or primary outcomes of the study.

Introduction

Most practitioners have experience in critical literature evaluation. Multiple item checklists are used to identify and evaluate important aspects of a study. While these multiple item lists can be helpful to the evaluator due to the great detail and number of specific points given to address within a study, they can also be time consuming and daunting for the practitioner. Health care professionals have a limited amount of time when deciding what articles to read and critically evaluate.

The purpose of this chapter is to reduce the burden of critical literature evaluation placed on the practitioner by introducing the Ten Major Considerations. The Ten Major Considerations are used to identify strengths and limitations in a study that have the greatest impact on the results/conclusions. Applying these considerations makes step three of the 5-Step Evidence-Based Medicine Process more efficient and user friendly for the busy practitioner.

Multiple Item Checklists

Often multiple item checklists are used as a teaching aid for students who are evaluating literature. An example of a multiple item checklist is provided at the end of this chapter. While these lengthy lists serve a purpose when orienting students to the critical literature evaluation process, they can be a barrier to the busy practitioner trying to assess studies in time-sensitive situations. Many items on multiple item checklists do not have a major impact on the study's overall validity nor do they shed much light on the reliability of the evidence provided by a study. In narrowing down these extensive checklists to the Ten Major Considerations, practitioners will find critical literature evaluation much more functional (see the table in **Figure 5.1** and also the "EBM Tool Kit" at the end of this book). The amount of time needed to thoroughly evaluate the integrity of an article is greatly reduced by using the Ten Major Considerations.

Ten Major Considerations

Once the Ten Major Considerations have been integrated into the practitioner's thought process, reading articles and determining their relevance become different. Major limitations that could have a significant impact on the study's integrity are taken into account, thus allowing the practitioner to recognize potential problems with the overall outcome of the study. By evaluating articles from this perspective, the practitioner is able to quickly identify the overall quality of evidence as well as which articles are worth reading.

Ten Major Considerations	Strength	Limitation
Power set/met?		
Dosage/treatment regimen appropriate?		
Length of study appropriate to show effect?		
Inclusion criteria adequate?		
Exclusion criteria adequate?		
Blinding present?		
Randomization resulted in similar groups?		
Biostatistical tests appropriate for type of data analyzed?		
Measurement(s) standard/validated/accepted practice?		
Author's conclusions are supported by the results?		

Figure 5.1: Ten Major Considerations

The Ten Major Considerations provide the practitioner with a concise and quick method to critically evaluate literature, a method that is much less daunting and time consuming compared to using a multiple item checklist. The Ten Major Considerations are presented in the table above and in detail below.

1. **Is power set and/or met?** Power is the ability of a study to detect statistically significant differences between treatment groups, when such a difference truly *does* exist. Once a study is verified as a randomized controlled trial, the practitioner can establish whether or not power was met. To determine this, the description for power should be found in the statistical section of most studies. When deciding whether or not a particular study met power, the practitioner should ask the following questions:

    ❑ What is power set at?

    ❑ How many patients are needed to meet power?

❑ What type of analysis is performed on the primary outcome measurements—per protocol or intent-to-treat?

❑ Does the number of patients used in the analysis meet the sample size required to meet power? If so, one should feel confident that enough patients are included to show a difference if one exists.

With practice, the above questions involving power should become "second nature" to the practitioner when looking at a study.

Example 5.1. Power Is Met

In a study conducted by Dahl et al.,[1] total sample size was based on estimated differences in average asthma exacerbation rate between two different treatments. "To detect a difference of 20% in the relative risk of exacerbations between salmeterol/fluticasone propionate (SFC) and formoterol/budesonide (FBC) combinations, at a two-sided $\alpha=0.05$ significance level with 90% power using the Normal approximation to the Poisson regression techniques, 525 patients per group were required." Intent-to-treat analyses were used for both primary and secondary outcome measures, with the primary outcome being rate of asthma exacerbations over a 6-month period. The final intent-to-treat analysis included 694 patients from the SFC group and 697 patients from the FBC group.

This example clearly states that 525 patients are needed in each treatment group to meet power for the primary outcome. This study undoubtedly met this requirement with both the SFC and FBC treatment groups, including well over 525 patients in their final analyses (n=694 and n=697, respectively). It is also important to determine whether or not a per protocol or intent-to-treat analysis was completed when determining power. A per protocol analysis requires knowing the number of patients that completed the study. An intent-to-treat analysis requires knowing the number of patients randomized into the study groups. Note that a modified intent-to-treat analysis includes specific criteria that must be met once a patient is randomized into the study (e.g., must have received at least one dose of the study drug or had at least one follow-up visit).

Understanding the importance of power in a study can be of great benefit for the practitioner trying to decipher what literature is worth reading in his or her limited time. In situations where power is not met or not calculated, the next question asked is: "Does a difference exist between treatment groups?" If a statistically significant difference is noted between treatment groups, the fact that the study did not meet power becomes less of a concern. If no statistically significant difference is found between treatment groups, a possibility exists that there were not enough people enrolled in the trial to detect a significant difference. This is a concern. Therefore, a clinician makes best use of time by reading trials that either *did* meet power or *did not* meet power but showed a statistically significant difference (potential type II error). See **Figure 5.2** for various power scenarios. For additional information on power, see Chapter 2: Basics for Interpretation.

Example 5.2. Power Is Not Met

In a trial performed by Gonzales et al.,[2] all study participants were randomized and all efficacy data was compared via intent-to-treat analysis. "A sample size of 335 participants per group was estimated as providing 90% power for a 2-tailed x^2 test with $\alpha=0.05$ for the comparison between varenicline and bupropion SR for the 4-week continuous abstinence rate based on an odds ratio

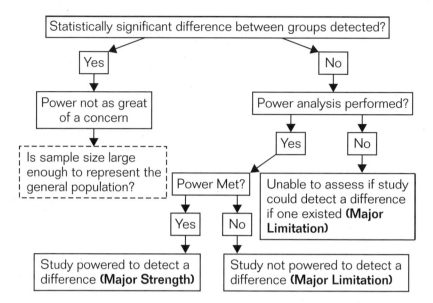

Figure 5.2: Power Scenarios

(OR) of 1.72 vs a bupropion SR response rate of 28.6%." Four-week continuous rates of abstinence between trial weeks 9 through 12 were confirmed via exhaled carbon monoxide. Varenicline (n=352) proved superior to placebo (n=344) (95% CI, 2.70–5.50; P<.001) and buproprion SR (n=329) (95% CI, 1.40–2.68; P<.001).

This example states that a sample size of 335 patients per group is needed to have 90% power. This trial failed to meet this goal with the buproprion SR group falling just short of the 335 patients required (n=329). While this study did not meet power, it is less of a concern because a statistically significant difference was seen in regards to the results. Varenicline proved to be superior to placebo and buproprion SR (P<0.001). In this case it would have been better for the trial to have met power, but since a statistically significant difference was still seen it was less of a concern and the potential for type II error was diminished.

2. **Are dosages and treatment regimens appropriate?** It is important to look at the dosage and/or treatment regimen used for each treatment group in a study. A potential major limitation can exist if a dosage and/or treatment regimen being used is not typically what is seen for the specific indication being addressed. This can help the practitioner recognize if sub- or supra-therapeutic dosing may have an effect on study results. It is also important to consider whether or not equivalent doses of study drugs are being compared. For instance, in a comparative trial evaluating cholesterol-lowering agents, one would not want simvastatin 80 mg to be compared to atorvastatin 10 mg. This comparison could potentially provide an advantage for one drug over the other and confound the results.

Example 5.3. Doses and Regimens Are Appropriate

In a study conducted by Manzoni et al.,[3] very low-birth-weight infants received fluconazole for prevention of fungal infections. For 2 weeks, infants were given 3 or 6 mg of fluconazole every third day; after the 2-week period, this became every other day. Normal saline was given on this same timetable to the placebo group. The study drug was administered intravenously through a catheter, if in use, or an orogastric tube.

In this example, a determination needed to be made in regards to appropriate dosing in the pediatric population. The main concern is safety of the dosage given in this study. Once safety is established, it is then appropriate to determine whether the dose of fluconazole used is similar to doses previously used for this indication. The *Lexi-Comp Pediatric Dosage Handbook* is a great resource for this example and helps the practitioner easily establish if the dosage being used in the study is suitable. The dosage in the above excerpt is a good example of a trial using an appropriate dosage regimen.

It is not always clear whether a dosage and/or regimen is appropriate when looking at a study that is investigating a non-FDA approved indication. Compendia such as *Lexi-Comp* and *Clinical Pharmacology* are helpful resources that refer to some non-FDA approved indications and doses. The safety of the dosage and/or treatment regimen is the primary concern. This can often be determined by reviewing other approved indications for the treatment in question to determine if dosages being used in the trial fall within these approved dosage ranges. In addition, some literature may address dosing for the particular non-FDA approved indication being studied.

Example 5.4. Doses and Regimens for a Non-FDA Approved Indication

Legro et al.[4] performed a trial examining clomiphene and metformin's efficacy in infertility associated with polycystic ovarian syndrome (PCOS). Metformin and clomiphene were begun concurrently upon study initiation. Patients received metformin 500 mg and clomiphene 50 mg, metformin 500 mg and matching clomiphene placebo, matching metformin placebo and clomiphene 50 mg, or just placebo. Subjects receiving metformin 500 mg increased their dosage to two tablets twice daily (maximum dose of four tablets) depending on their tolerability of the drug. Subjects randomized to clomiphene were given one 50-mg clomiphene tablet to be taken for 5 days beginning on the third day of menses. Documentation of adequate ovulation determined whether clomiphene dosage should be maintained. A dosage increase of one additional 50-mg tablet per day was made in patients with no response or minimal response to clomiphene.

In cases where a study is evaluating a non-FDA approved indication like the above example for metformin and polycystic ovarian syndrome (PCOS), the first concern should be for the safety of the particular dosage regimen in patients. *Lexi-Comp* and *Clinical Pharmacology* are resources that may include recommended dosing for non-FDA approved indications. If unable to confirm appropriate dosing using these resources, the practitioner's next step is to ensure dosing is within appropriate ranges seen in indications in which the medication has been approved. In this case, the non-FDA approved dose for metformin in PCOS is listed in *Clinical Pharmacology* as 500 mg three times daily. While the above study uses a higher dosage for PCOS than reported in *Clinical Pharmacology* (two 500-mg tablets twice daily), it is still considered appropriate because it is not out of range when looking at an FDA-approved indication for metformin such as diabetes.

3. **Is the length of the study appropriate to show effect?**
    A study conducted for an inadequate length of time can result in no treatment effect seen when there really is potential for an effect. In most situations, the concern will be whether or not the trial was conducted for a long enough period of time. For instance, some antidepressant medications such as selective serotonin reuptake inhibitors (SSRIs) require 4–6 weeks to see any effect or improvement in patients. A study involving these agents only lasting 3 weeks may not be an adequate amount of time to show any significant differences in efficacy.

4.   **Are inclusion criteria adequate?** Inclusion criteria are developed primarily to ensure the correct patient population is used to determine efficacy. To participate in any well-designed study, subjects must meet certain criteria before being approved for inclusion in a trial. Investigators identify specific parameters such as age, disease state and/or stage of disease state, sex, treatment history, and other medical conditions that may influence trial results. When inclusion criteria are not properly defined, the possibility exists that a study may be using patients not representative of the population that the investigators intended to treat. Correctly selecting the inclusion criteria for a trial can have a large impact on whether or not the study is clinically relevant to the question being asked. Choosing to include patients outside the target disease state or whose demographics are not appropriate for the desired population may have an impact on the results of the study. In these cases, clinical judgment must be used to determine the extent of the effect.

Example 5.5. Inclusion Criteria

Tfelt-Hansen and associates[5] conducted a study comparing sumatriptan versus rizatriptan in acute treatment of migraine. Patients who met proper criteria for migraine with or without aura as determined by the International Headache Society (IHS) were enrolled in the trial. Subjects were required to be in good health and to have had at least a 6-month history of migraines, experiencing between one and eight attacks per month. Enrolled subjects were both male and female aged 18–65 years.

When determining whether or not inclusion criteria are appropriate, it is important to keep in mind why criteria are developed in the first place. Trial investigators must ensure that the correct patient population is used to determine efficacy, otherwise a study may be evaluating a population that is not representative of the one they set out to treat. In the example shown above, it was the investigator's intent to compare two migraine medications within the same class and the effect they had on patients with acute migraine. The inclusion criteria developed in this example resulted in a patient population appropriate for the study. Practitioners who are evaluating inclusion criteria should always ask whether the patient population enrolled is representative of the population they intend to treat.

When evaluating a study for adequate inclusion criteria, the practitioner should also identify any inclusion criteria not mentioned that would be important to the specific trial. If certain inclusion criteria are identified as absent, the practitioner must assess whether or not there is a potential effect on the results due to this deficit.

5.   **Are exclusion criteria adequate?** Patient safety is the primary focus when establishing exclusion criteria. This is the investigator's opportunity to exclude any patients who may be at risk for increased adverse events and other safety issues by participating in the trial. Just as investigators determine specific parameters or guidelines to establish those patients to be included in a trial, parameters are also established for patients who will be excluded because of safety reasons. Factors such as co-morbid conditions and concurrent medications that have the possibility of increasing the risk of adverse events are taken into consideration.

Exclusion criteria not only ensure safety in a study but guard against inclusion of patients who could potentially decrease one's ability to determine if results are due to the study treatment or another factor. Below are a few examples of these potential factors:

❑ Previous exposure to the study treatment/similar treatment within 6 months of the study
❑ Any current medication use that could bias the results
❑ Certain co-morbid conditions and/or disease states
❑ Previous procedures affecting the study drug or disease state in question

It is also important to identify instances when exclusion criteria are too restrictive, thus creating a study less relevant to the specific patient population requiring treatment.

Example 5.6. Exclusion Criteria

A multi-center trial to assess low-dose orlistat effects on body weight of mild to moderately overweight individuals was conducted by Anderson et al. Subjects were excluded if they had any of the following: prior weight loss surgery, prior weight loss of 3 kg or more in the past 3 months, use of any medications that have an effect on weight loss within the past 6 months, bulimia and/or laxative abuse, untreated thyroid disease, history within the past 6 months of CABG or angioplasty procedure with cardiovascular disease, diabetes currently controlled by medication, recent smoking cessation within last 6 months, and use of any medications that interact with orlistat. Pregnant or breastfeeding women were not included.

When determining whether a study has selected appropriate exclusion criteria, emphasis is placed on patient safety. It is the investigator's job to make sure all patients who potentially could be safety risks are excluded from the trial. Many times this means learning more about the medication being studied and its adverse effects. The above exclusion criteria in the orlistat trial adequately addressed safety concerns such as drug interactions, pregnancy, and cardiovascular considerations.

The above trial also accounted for concurrent medications and/or underlying disease states that could have impacted the results. For instance, investigators excluded patients with untreated thyroid disease such as hypothyroidism or any use of pharmacological agents within the last 6 months affecting body weight. With the exclusion of these factors, the investigators decreased the possibility that results of the trial would show anything but the effect orlistat had on weight loss of patients enrolled in the study.

Investigators may fail to identify all appropriate exclusion criteria. If certain exclusion criteria were left out, any potential effect this had on the study results should be assessed.

Example 5.7. Exclusion Criteria Are Not Adequate

In a study conducted by Kolodony and colleagues,[7] treatments for acute migraine were compared. Study participants were excluded from the trial if they used any of the following drugs: propranolol, methylsergide, and monoamine oxidase inhibitors. The use of standard antimigraine prophylactic medications was allowed except for the use of NSAIDs, daily analgesics, or propranolol. Pregnant or lactating women were not eligible for inclusion into the study.

The above study defined many exclusion criteria that were appropriate for ensuring the safety of trial participants when using the triptan medications. Unfortunately, the authors neglected one major safety issue with the triptan medications: cardiovascular concerns. Serotonin receptor agonists, such as the triptans, may increase the potential for cardiovascular side effects; this should be addressed within the exclusion criteria. When evaluating the adequacy of exclusion criteria, the practitioner should be familiar with all safety concerns of the particular medication or treatment being studied.

6.   **Is the study blinded?** An adequately blinded study guards against investigator and subject bias. Typically, one would like to see double-blinded studies because they attempt to prevent the largest degree of investigator or patient bias in a trial. In single-blinded studies (where either the investigator or patient is not blinded to the intervention), there is a greater chance for bias to confound the results.

The exact method of blinding is seldom explained in the article. Rather, a statement that the study was blinded is usually seen. The practitioner should question whether there were any potential barriers to successfully blinding a particular drug. For instance, a peculiar smell or taste characteristic of the study drug should also be reproduced for the control(s) to maintain blinding. That smell or taste in some cases can be masked for the study drug. In either situation, an explanation of how this was handled should be provided. If there is no explanation, the practitioner must assume the issue was not addressed. Blinding is considered a major limitation when this occurs; however, the practitioner still needs to assess whether that major limitation had any effect on the overall results/conclusions.

Example 5.8. Blinding

A double-blind, placebo-controlled trial in patients with pulmonary hypertension performed by Galie et al.[8] used a stratified central-randomization scheme to allocate patients to their four respective treatment groups (sildenafil 20, 40, or 80 mg or placebo). Dose escalation took place for the first 7 days of the study for those patients assigned to the 80-mg treatment group. They received 40 mg three times daily for 7 days and then moved up to 80 mg three times daily. Dummy dose escalation was also performed for the other three treatment groups during the first 7 days.

Although the trial described above was double blinded and took measures to conceal dose escalation in the sildenafil 80-mg treatment group, there is still potential for blinding to be flawed. Sildenafil's side effect profile includes incidence of penile erection in male patients, which could potentially cause patients to become unblinded to their respective treatment groups. The authors do not address this potential weakness in the blinding of the study.

7.   **Did randomization result in similar groups?** When randomization is successful, each patient has an equal chance of being assigned to one treatment group versus the other(s). Even more critical is that the trial ends up with very similar groups demographically following randomization. If a significant disparity is found between treatment groups, there is concern about whether the results observed are due to the study drug or a difference that was present between groups from the start. For instance, in a clinical trial evaluating the efficacy of an asthma medication, it is important that a similar number of smokers are randomized to each treatment group. If groups are dissimilar, the results seen may not accurately depict the medication's efficacy and may potentially be due to a lower or higher number of smokers being randomized to a particular group.

The demographics table in a study is useful for confirming similar treatment groups. When dissimilarities are found, it is important to question what impact or clinical relevance the dissimilarity could have had on the results. For instance, disease states often have many levels of severity. If one treatment group has more severe patients than the other after randomization, the drug's efficacy may be falsely reported as reduced in that group compared to the group with less severe patients. The practitioner must also be aware of any additional demographic information that should have been collected or discussed but was not. If this occurs, it is important to question what impact this discrepancy may have had on the results.

Example 5.9. Similar Groups after Randomization and Statistics

A modified table below illustrates baseline characteristics seen in a trial evaluating the effects on fracture rate of continuing or stopping alendronate after 5 years of treatment by Black et al.:[9]

Characteristics	(n=437) Placebo	(5 mg/d) (n=329) Alendronate	(10 mg/d) (n=333) Alendronate	P Value
Body mass index, mean (SD)	25.8 (4.3)	25.7 (4.2)	25.9 (4.5)	.05
Race White	421 (96.3)	322 (97.9)	327 (98.2)	.22
Other	16 (3.7)	7 (2.1)	6 (1.8)	.22
Walk for exercise	244 (57.0)	189 (58.7)	203 (61.9)	.40
Fall in last 12 mo.	105 (24.2)	80 (24.4)	71 (21.6)	
History of clinical fracture (>45 years old)	260 (59.5)	196 (59.6)	204 (61.3)	.86
Current alendronate use	341 (78.0)	275 (83.6)	262 (78.7)	.13

The above example demonstrates how some trials display demographic data. Statistics were run on the demographic data above, helping the practitioner to detect any significant differences seen in baseline characteristics after randomization. When studies provide statistical information on baseline data, it makes identifying significant differences much easier. For instance, if p-values were not provided, one might question whether or not a significant difference was seen. No significant differences were seen in the above example. If a significant difference had been seen, the practitioner should question what impact the difference would have had on the results of the trial.

Example 5.10. Similar Groups after Randomization and No Demographic Table

In a study conducted by Anderson et al.,[6] "the baseline demographics of the placebo and orlistat groups were similar. Of the 378 subjects, 94.4% were female (n=357), 89.2% were white (n=337), average ($\pm$SD) age was 46.2 $\pm$ 11.41 years, baseline weight was 72.8 $\pm$ 6.97 kg, and BMI was 26.8 $\pm$ 0.96 kg/m^2."

Not all studies will address the similarity of demographics among treatment groups after randomization in the same way. For instance, the above example is from a trial that just briefly mentioned groups were similar in the text of the article. No chart or statistics were given. In these cases, the practitioner must decide whether this major consideration was adequately addressed and what impact may be seen on the results.

Statistical tests are not always performed on demographic information in a trial (see **Example 5.10**). This means the practitioner is not always provided with information about whether statistically significant differences are seen between each group's demographic characteristics. In these instances, a judgment call must be made by the practitioner to determine if any differences exist that may impact the results.

Example 5.11. Similar Groups after Randomization and No Statistics

An open-label, parallel group, randomized controlled trial by Farmer et al.[10] evaluated the impact of self monitoring of blood glucose in patients with non-insulin treated diabetes:

Characteristics	Control Group	Less Intensive Self-Monitoring Group	More Intensive Self-Monitoring Group
Mean (SD) age (years)	66.3 (10.2)	65.2 (10.6)	65.5 (9.9)
Men	85 (55.9)	88 (58.7)	87 (57.6)
Median (interquartile range) duration (years) of diabetes	3 (2–6)	3 (2–7)	3 (2–6)
Treatment			
Diet only	44 (28.9)	39 (26.0)	41 (27.2)
Monotherapy	57 (37.5)	58 (38.7)	58 (38.4)
Combined oral therapy	51 (33.6)	53 (35.3)	52 (34.4)
Use of blood glucose meter			
Not using	104 (68.4)	110 (73.3)	102 (67.5)
Using once weekly or less	48 (31.6)	40 (26.7)	49 (32.5)
Mean (SD) hemoglobin A_{1c} (%)	7.49 (1.09)	7.41 (1.02)	7.53 (1.12)

> Although a chart was provided in this study to illustrate baseline characteristics, the table was not analyzed for statistically significant differences seen. In these instances, the practitioner must use clinical judgment to determine if any demographic information appears to be significantly different. If something is identified, the next step is questioning what effect that difference will have on results.

When analyzing data using a per protocol analysis, one should ensure that groups are similar at the end of the study. A per protocol analysis utilizes the results seen in each of the treatment groups at the completion of a study. Patients withdraw from studies for various reasons, which can result in different groups at the end of the trial. When evaluating a study using a per protocol analysis, the evaluator should attempt to determine if the groups are similar at completion of the trial. When a difference between groups occurs at the end of a study, it is important to question what impact or clinical relevance the dissimilarity may have on results.

Finally, it is important to remember that even a well planned and adequately conducted randomization can fail and result in dissimilar groups. In this instance, the practitioner evaluating the study must determine if these differences have any significant impact on the results.

8. **Are appropriate statistical tests used for type(s) of data analyzed?** The reader must determine if the appropriate statistical test was used for the type of data analyzed. This particular consideration tends to create the most difficulty for the practitioner. Using the incorrect statistical test for the type of data analyzed can have serious negative impact on the results, making them impossible to interpret accurately. When the incorrect statistical test is used for the type of data analyzed, the results should not be trusted unless the authors have provided an adequate

explanation why the tests in question were used. Luckily for the practitioner, this determination does not have to be such a tedious and puzzling process. When one is equipped with the right tools, identifying the correct statistical test in a trial can be straightforward. A good understanding of the different types of data (nominal, ordinal, interval, and ratio) used in trials and access to an appropriate statistical test reference is all that is necessary. A chart detailing when certain statistical tests should or should not be used is found in Chapter 2: Basics for Interpretation, Figure 2.13.

9.   **Are evaluation measurements standard, validated, or accepted practice?** When choosing how to accurately measure the primary outcome of a study, the investigators should select evaluation measurements that are validated or accepted in practice. In addition, it is important to verify that the outcome measure being used is relevant to the disease state in question. For instance, weight loss should not be used as a primary outcome measure in a trial investigating the efficacy of an oral diabetic agent in lowering blood glucose levels.

Example 5.12. Appropriate Evaluation Tool

In a trial performed by Sastry and associates,[11] the efficacy of sildenafil versus placebo for primary pulmonary hypertension was studied. The Naughton protocol was used to help evaluate the primary endpoint of the study, which was "change in exercise time on treadmill."

It is important to establish the appropriateness of both the primary outcome of a study as well as the evaluation tool used to measure that primary outcome. Determining whether an outcome measure and/or evaluation tool is validated or accepted in practice can be done in a variety of different ways. For instance, the above example uses "change in exercise time on treadmill" as the primary outcome measure and the Naughton protocol as the evaluation tool. A quick literature search confirms that both this outcome measure and evaluation tool are frequently used when looking at the disease state of primary pulmonary hypertension. Also, the Naughton protocol is described in many clinical exercise physiology textbooks as being an approved method for treadmill tests. Therefore, both the outcome measure and tool are validated and accepted methods in practice.

Even if the results of a study are statistically significant, they are questionable and potentially not applicable if an inappropriate evaluation method is used to measure the primary outcome.

If you are unfamiliar with an outcome measure or test being used in a particular study, further investigation is warranted. When the measurement or test in question is referenced, the practitioner can go to the reference cited to determine if the measurement or test has been validated and/or is an accepted practice. In cases where the evaluation tool in question has not been referenced, the following questions may be asked when determining the appropriateness of the outcome measure or test.

❑ Do studies looking at this same outcome use this particular evaluation tool?

❑ Is this method or test validated?

❑ Does the evaluation method being used measure something that is clinically relevant to the disease state or medication being studied?

❑ Is this a new trend being used to evaluate this specific outcome?

10.   **Are author's conclusions supported by the results?** Finally, results and/or primary outcomes seen in studies must support the conclusions made by the authors of those articles. There should be concern when conclusions are drawn by study investigators that do not seem to coincide with the results reported in a trial. This kind of disparity between the results of a study and the conclusion may indicate investigator bias and should be questioned.

Summary

While multiple item checklists can be a very detailed and specific tool for introducing critical literature evaluation, it is unrealistic to believe this is the most efficient way to evaluate literature for the busy practitioner. Identification of the Ten Major Considerations and how they impact the results allows the practitioner to not only evaluate literature effectively but also reduce the amount of time spent performing this task. Integration of these considerations into the practitioner's thought process can change the approach by which articles are read and evaluated. This will also aid the practitioner in determining what articles are worthy of his or her limited time.

References

1.   Dahl R, Chuchalin A, Gor D, et al. EXCEL: A randomized trial comparing salmeterol/fluticasone propionate and formoterol/budesonide combinations in adults with persistent asthma. *Respiratory Medicine.* 2006; 100:1152–1162.

2.   Gonzales D, Rennard SI, Nides M, et al. Varenicline, an $\alpha 4\beta 2$ nicotinic acetylcholine receptor partial agonist, vs sustained-release bupropion and placebo for smoking cessation, a randomized controlled trial. *JAMA.* 2006; 296:47–55.

3. Manzoni P, Stolfi I, Pugni L, et al. A multicenter, random-ized trial of prophylactic fluconazole in preterm neonates. *N Engl J Med.* 2007; 356:2483–2495.

4. Legro RS, Barnhart HX, Schlaff WD, et al. Clomiphene, metformin, or both for infertility in the polycystic ovary syndrome. *N Engl J Med.* 2007; 356:551–566.

5. Tfelt-Hansen P, Teall J, Rodriguez F, et al. Oral rizatriptan versus oral sumatriptan: A direct comparative study in the acute treatment of migraine. *Headache.* 1998; 38:748–755.

6. Anderson J, Schwartz S, Hauptman J, et al. Low-dose orlistat effects on body weight of mildly to moderately overweight individuals: a 16 week, double-blind, placebo-controlled trial. *Ann Pharmacother.* 2006; 40:1717–1723.

7. Kolodony A, Polis A, Battisti WP, et al. Comparison of rizatriptan 5 mg and 10 mg tablets and sumatriptan 25 mg and 50 mg tablets. *Cephalalgia.* 2004; 24:540–546.

8. Galie N, Ghofrani H, Torbicki A, et al. Sildenafil citrate therapy for pulmonary arterial hypertension. *N Engl J Med.* 2005; 353:2148–2157.

9. Black D, Schwartz A, Ensrud K, et al. Effects of continu-ing or stopping alendronate after 5 years of treatment. The fracture intervention trial long-term extension (FLEX): a randomized trial. *JAMA.* 2006; 296:2927–2938.

10. Farmer A, Wade A, Goyder E, et al. Impact of self moni-toring of blood glucose in the management of patients with non-insulin treated diabetes: open parallel group randomized trial. *BMJ.* 2007; 335:132–139.

11. Sastry BK, Narasimhan C, Reddy NK, et al. Clinical effi-cacy of sildenafil in primary pulmonary hypertension: a randomized, placebo-controlled, double-blind, crossover study. *J Am Coll Cardiol.* 2004; 43:1149–1153.

Evaluation of Primary Literature: Multi-item Checklist

Article Title: _____

Checklist Item	Y/N	S/W	Justification
1. Is the journal peer-reviewed?			
2. Is title biased?			
3. Are investigators considered reliable and was study conducted in a reputable medical center or university teaching hospital? If not, is location adequate for application of good scientific experimental method?			
4. Are objectives and/or hypothesis (i.e., purpose) clearly defined?			
5. Were inclusion criteria appropriate for the purposes of the study?			
6. Were exclusion criteria appropriate for the purposes of the study?			
7. In addition to inclusion/exclusion criteria, was adequate pertinent patient information provided (e.g., disease severity, demographics, previous treatment failure, smoking status, lifestyle habits, etc.)?			
8. Were recruitment methods targeted toward persons likely to be representative of applicable population?			
9. Was trial prospective or retrospective?	X	X	
10. Was a control established?			
11. If so, was type of control appropriate?			
12. Were study drug and controls allocated randomly? (If given, what method was used?)			
13. Were group characteristics similar after randomization? If possible to determine, was the similarity of characteristics maintained throughout study completion, i.e., after dropouts?			
14. Was study blinded and, if so, were blinding techniques appropriate?			
15. Were drug doses and regimens appropriate (e.g., within known therapeutic ranges, safe, proper interval, equally effective doses when active drugs compared)?			
16. Was treatment duration adequate for assessing effect?			

Checklist Item	Y/N	S/W	Justification
17. Were any drugs used concurrently? Was concurrent drug use discussed?			
18. Were outcome measurements validated or accepted practice?			
19. Were steps taken to decrease inter-rater variability?			
20. Did authors discuss any factors or influences that may have affected results of outcome measures? Were there additional sources of bias noted?			
21. Were there any problems in reporting or accuracy of results (e.g., did text and table/graph data agree, any missing data)?			
22. Were side effects reported?			
23. Were type, severity, and incidence of side effects reported?			
24. Were the number of dropouts reported?			
25. Were precise reasons for dropouts discussed?			
26. Was a per protocol or an intent-to-treat analysis used?	XXX	XXX	
27. How many subjects were enrolled?	XXX	XXX	
28. How many subjects were included in final statistical analysis?	XXX	XXX	
29. Was a power calculation performed?			
30. If a power calculation was performed, was power met at study end?			
31. Were all statistical tests used appropriate for types of data (nominal, ordinal, or interval)?			
32. Are conclusions and recommendations consistent with results obtained?			
33. Does article provide a reference list to verify footnoted citations?			

Other strengths/weakness specific to this article

1.

2.

3.

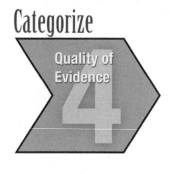

Categorize

Chapter 6

Categorize Quality of Evidence

Patrick J. Bryant

Step 4 – Categorize Quality of Evidence

After completing the critical evaluation of a specific trial, the practitioner needs to categorize the quality of evidence. This fourth step is the bridge between performing a critical literature evaluation and developing a recommendation.

Key Idea

Categorizing the quality of evidence is the bridge between performing a critical literature evaluation and developing a recommendation with justifications.

Quality of evidence is determined by evaluating specific study design characteristics and key study attributes (see **Figure 6.1**).

QUALITY OF EVIDENCE   =

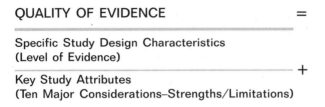

$$\frac{\text{Specific Study Design Characteristics (Level of Evidence)}}{\text{Key Study Attributes (Ten Major Considerations–Strengths/Limitations)}} +$$

Figure 6.1: Quality of Evidence Equation

For instance, a randomization scheme, comparison group, and adequate sample size are specific study design characteristics. In addition, key attributes that strengthen or weaken the basic study design are considered.

Key Idea

The quality of evidence equation includes specific study design characteristics and key study attributes that determine the overall quality of evidence for a particular study.

These key attributes are represented by the Ten Major Considerations that were previously used to critically evaluate articles (see Chapter 5: Evaluate Literature). Both components of the quality of evidence equation (specific study design characteristics and key study attributes) are required for an accurate categorization of the quality of evidence.

Levels of Evidence—Specific Study Design Characteristics

A ranking system referred to as levels of evidence is utilized to categorize studies based on quality of design.

Key Idea

The level of evidence for a study categorizes the overall study design quality.

Several methods exist to categorize a study's level of evidence.[1-8] The method used in this chapter provides a simple, straightforward, and logical approach. Originally described by Drs. Deborah Cook and Gordon Guyatt, this method incorporates a modified approach.[9] The process is based on four specific study design characteristics that assist in categorizing studies by their respective levels of evidence. These specific study design characteristics are

1. Interventional or observational study design

2. Controlled or non-controlled study design

3. Randomized or non-randomized study design

4. Power set/met or not set/met for the study design

Using this method, a study is assigned Levels I through V, with Level I representing the highest level of study design quality (see table in **Figure 6.2**).

Level of Evidence	Study Design Characteristics	Quality of Design
Level I	Interventional Randomized Controlled Trials with Meeting Power	*****
Level II	Interventional Randomized Controlled Trials with Not Meeting Power	****
Level III	Observational Prospective Trials	***
Level IV	Observational Retrospective Trials	**
Level V	Case Studies, Case Series, and Case Reports	*

Figure 6.2: Levels of Evidence – Study Design Characteristics and Quality of Study Design

Key Idea

Using the level of evidence ranking system, a study is assigned one of five categories, Level I through Level V; Level I represents the highest level of study design quality.

Example 6.1. Relationship Between Study Design Characteristics and Levels of Evidence

A randomized, controlled trial comparing two different drugs for use in irritable bowel syndrome could be

- **Level I** if powered to show a difference if one really existed.

- **Level II** if power is not met or not initially set to show a difference if one existed.

Studies used to observe changes such as incidence of constipation versus diarrhea associated with irritable bowel syndrome without intervention in a population of patients over time could be

- **Level III** if a prospective observational study design is used.

- **Level IV** if a retrospective observational study design is used.

A testimonial of how well stress reduction exercises reduce irritable bowel symptoms in a single patient or series of patients would be considered

- **Level V** since no randomization scheme, control group, or set power exists.

The progression from Level I to Level V represents a decrease in quality of study design and, therefore, reliability of results provided by that particular trial. As the evidence used to develop a recommendation decreases in quality (Level I going to Level V), the overall strength of that recommendation also decreases. In other words, Level I evidence represents the highest possible level of study design quality; Level V evidence represents the lowest level of study design quality. Recommendations are developed from the highest level of evidence available. When no evidence exists, recommendations are made based on experience which can overestimate efficacy and underestimate safety risks.

Five Questions to Ask

Five questions are asked to determine existence of these specific study design characteristics within a particular trial. Diagrams are provided to help illustrate the differences between the five levels of evidence (**Figures 6.3–6.7**).

Key Idea

Five questions are asked and answered to determine the existence of specific study design characteristics within a study:

1. Does the study have an intervention or is it strictly observational?

2. Does the study have a control group?

3. Does the observational study look forward or backward in time (prospective or retrospective)?

4. Is the study randomized?

5. If the study is a randomized and controlled trial, is power met?

Question #1: Does the study have an intervention or is it strictly observational? In other words, are patients being assigned a specific therapy or intervention?

> **Level I and Level II** evidence are represented by trials with an *interventional* study design (see **Figure 6.3**). The investigators are assigning a specific intervention to each subject. For instance, a trial to identify the effects of an anti-diabetic agent would require a group of subjects to be given the intervention (drug).

> **Levels III and IV** evidence are represented by trials with an *observational* study design. In observational trials, investiga-

tors are merely observing the subjects and no intervention is being assigned. Subjects are chosen based on presence or absence of specific characteristics. A trial observing what complications occur to diabetic patients with lack of long-term glycemic control versus diabetic patients with long-term glycemic control is considered an observational trial.

Level V evidence is represented by trials with either an *interventional* or *observational* study design.

Note that trials utilizing an interventional study design represent the higher levels of evidence (Levels I, II). Those trials utilizing an observational study design represent a lower level of evidence (Level III, IV), and the trial design representing the lowest level of evidence is Level V. The progression from Level I to Level V evidence represents a decrease in quality of trial design and, therefore, reliability of results provided by that particular trial. A decrease in quality and reliability of evidence corresponds to a decrease in overall strength of the recommendation being developed.

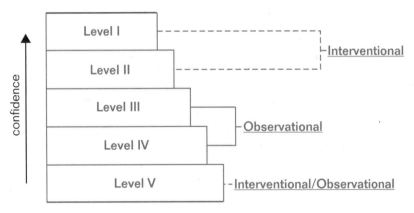

Figure 6.3: Levels of Evidence – Interventional versus Observational Study Design

Key Idea

The strength of a recommendation is weakened when evidence of low quality and reliability is used.

Question #2: Does the study have a control group?

Level I and Level II evidence are represented by trials with a *control* group (see **Figure 6.4**). Control groups provide a comparison to ensure that changes seen in the intervention group are due to something other than chance.

Level III and Level IV evidence are also represented by trials with a *control* group. This control group can be either prospective or retrospective in nature. As with interventional trials, the control group serves as a way to ensure that changes seen in the study group are due to something other than chance.

Level V evidence is represented by trials without a control group. Without a control group, there is no way to confirm that changes seen in a subject or group of subjects are due to something other than chance. Essentially, Level V trials are equivalent to personal testimonials. Level V trials typically consist of a single-case study, case series, and/or case report.

Note that trials containing a control group represent the higher levels of evidence (Levels I through IV). Those trials containing no control group represent the lowest level of evidence (Level V). The progression from Level I to Level V evidence represents a decrease in the quality of the trial design and, therefore, reliability of the results provided by that particular trial. Without high quality and reliabile evidence, the strength of the recommendation is compromised.

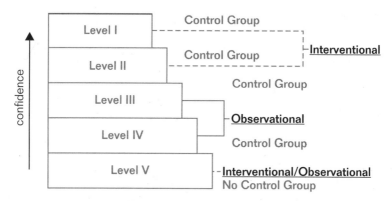

Figure 6.4: Levels of Evidence – Control Group versus No Control Group Study Design

Question #3: Does the observational study look forward or backward in time (prospective or retrospective)?

Level III evidence is represented by observational trials that *look forward* in time using prospective cohort groups of subjects (see **Figure 6.5**). In prospective observational trials, the investigators define the disease and the predicted variables prior to the onset of disease. Subjects are chosen based on specific characteristics (e.g., smoking) and followed forward in time to observe the development of a specific outcome (e.g., lung cancer). For a more detailed description of prospective observational trials, see Chapter 2: Basics for Interpretation.

Example 6.2. Level III Prospective Observational Trial

Level III evidence is represented by a trial such as the Harvard Nurse's Health Study II that is considered one of the most significant studies conducted on the health of women. This study has been following nurses and the progression of their health since 1989. An example of the results includes the long-term effect of moderate alcohol consumption on the nurse's cognitive function. In this analysis, cognitive function was monitored over time in nurses consuming moderate quantities of alcohol. A similar group of nurses who were not consuming alcohol were followed simultaneously over the same time period and represent the *prospective cohort* comparison group.

Level IV evidence is represented by observational trials that *look back* in time using retrospective cohort or case control groups. For instance, investigators will examine the data for a group of subjects with a diagnosis of lung cancer and examine smoking history of the group to determine if an association exists between smoking and development of lung cancer. For a more detailed description of retrospective observational trials, see Chapter 2: Basics for Interpretation.

> ## Example 6.3. Level IV Retrospective Observational Trial
>
> An observational study is designed to examine the differences in lifestyle between patients that have developed esophageal cancer versus those who have not developed this disease. The investigators randomly select charts from an institution's medical records of patients who developed esophageal cancer. Various characteristics such as lifestyle are identified that may have led to the development of the esophageal cancer such as a consistent diet of extremely spicy foods.

Note that observational trials using a *prospective design* represent a higher level of evidence (Level III) than trials containing a *retrospective design,* which represent a lower level of evidence (Level IV). Trials using a prospective design have less potential for bias interfering with the results than those with a retrospective design. The progression from Level III to Level IV evidence represents a decrease in quality of the trial design and, therefore, reliability of results provided by that particular trial. Only high quality and reliable evidence can provide a strong recommendation.

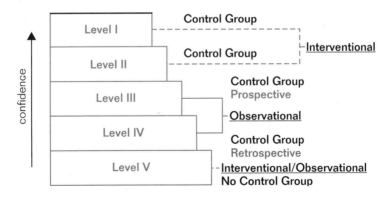

Figure 6.5: Levels of Evidence – Prospective versus Retrospective Observational Study Design

Question #4: Is the study randomized?

Level I and Level II trials utilize a *randomization scheme* to assign patients to study groups (see **Figure 6.6**). Randomization, when done correctly, ensures each subject has an equal chance of being assigned to either of the study groups. The result of a trial with a successful randomization scheme has study groups with similar demographic characteristics following the randomization process; differences in an outcome measure between groups at the end of the study are more likely attributable to the intervention.

Level III, Level IV, and Level V trials do not utilize a randomization scheme to assign patients into various groups. Rather, subjects to be entered into the trial can be chosen at random. For instance, out of a potential subject pool of 500, the investigators randomly select 300 subjects for the study. (See **Example 6.4**)

Example 6.4. Random Selection of Subjects for Observational Trials

A prospective observational trial (Level III) examining the long-term effects of smoking would include subjects randomly selected from a pool of subjects with a history of smoking. These patients are followed forward in time to observe the development of specific outcomes (e.g., lung cancer).

Note that trials utilizing a randomization scheme to assign patients to study groups represent the higher level of evidence (Level I and Level II). Those trials utilizing no randomization scheme represent the lower levels of evidence (Levels III, IV, and V). A successful randomization scheme assures that each patient has an equal opportunity of being assigned to one group versus another, and this should result in demographically similar groups. Changes noted in the study results can then be attributed to something other than starting out with dissimilar groups. The progression from Level I to Level V evidence represents a decrease in quality of the trial design and, therefore, reliability of results provided by that particular trial. The strength of the recommendation is decreased when the quality and reliability of the evidence is low.

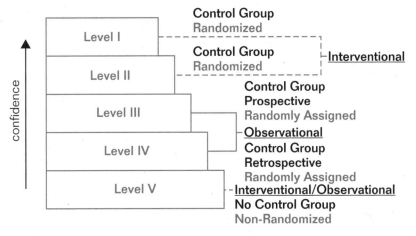

Figure 6.6: Levels of Evidence – Randomized or Non-Randomized Study Design

Question #5: If the study is an interventional randomized and controlled trial, is power met?

Level I evidence is represented by trials where power *is set and met* (see **Figure 6.7** and also the "EBM Tool Kit" at the end of this book). In these trials, the sample size is adequate to show a difference between study groups, if a difference really exists.

Level II evidence is represented by trials where power *is set and not met* or power *is not set* or not mentioned at all. Power especially becomes important when no statistically significant difference is found between the treatment groups. In this situation, a difference between treatment groups may have been observed if additional patients were enrolled to meet power. For this reason, no definitive conclusion can be made that the groups are similar.

Note that trials where power is set and met represent the higher level of evidence (Level I). Those trials where power is set and not met or not mentioned represent the lower level of evidence (Level II). As pointed out in Chapter 2: Basics for Interpretation, power is used to determine an adequate sample size that will show a difference between treatment groups, if a difference really exists. The progression from Level I to Level II evidence represents a decrease in quality of the trial design and, therefore, reliability of results provided by that particular trial. Higher quality and reliability of evidence is associated with an overall increase in strength of the recommendation.

Please refer to the table in **Figure 6.8** for a summary of specific study design characteristics for each level of evidence. In addition, this table illustrates the degree of confidence associated with each level of evidence.

Ten Major Considerations—Key Study Attributes

As discussed earlier, the second part of the quality of evidence equation is the consideration of *key study attributes* that strengthen or weaken the basic study design (refer back to Figure 6.1). These key study attributes are represented by the Ten Major Considerations used to critically evaluate an article (see Chapter 5: Evaluate Literature).

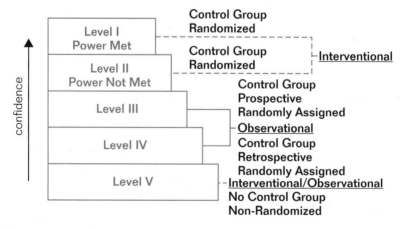

Figure 6.7: Levels of Evidence – Power Met versus Power Not Met Study Design

Level of Evidence	Interventional versus Observational (I and/or O)	Control Group (Yes/No)	Prospective versus Retrospective (P or R)	Randomized (Yes/No)	Power Met (Yes/No)	Confidence
Level I	I	Y	P	Y	Y	+++++
Level II	I	Y	P	Y	N	++++
Level III	O	Y	P	N*	-	+++
Level IV	O	Y	R	N*	-	++
Level V	I/O	N	P/R	N	-	+

* Randomly assigned to study, but not to study groups.

Figure 6.8: Levels of Evidence – Summary of Specific Study Design Characteristics by Level of Evidence

In addition to the level of evidence, the second component of quality of the evidence equation is consideration of key study attributes. These key study attributes are represented by the Ten Major Considerations used to critically evaluate an article. Presence of these key study attributes contributes to strengthening the quality of the study's design.

If one of the Ten Major Considerations (key study attribute) is present in the study, that attribute is considered a major strength (see table in **Figure 6.9**). However, if that same major consideration or key study attribute is absent or lacking, a major limitation is determined to exist for that study.

Ten Major Considerations	Strength	Limitation
Power set/met?		
Dosage/treatment regimen appropriate?		
Length of study appropriate to show effect?		
Inclusion criteria adequate?		
Exclusion criteria adequate?		
Blinding present?		
Randomization resulted in similar groups?		
Biostatistical tests appropriate for type of data analyzed?		
Measurement(s) standard/validated/accepted practice?		
Author's conclusions are supported by the results?		

Figure 6.9: Ten Major Considerations

Key Idea

Level I evidence with minor limitations represents the highest quality of evidence. A Level V study—with all Ten Major Considerations being limitations—is considered the lowest quality of evidence.

The next question to ask when a major limitation is identified is whether this limitation appears to have an effect on the overall study results. *If the answer is yes to that question, then the overall quality of that trial is lessened, even though the level of evidence remains the same.*

Example 6.5. Major Limitation: Impact versus No Impact on Study Results

A Level I trial has a major limitation of randomization not resulting in similar groups. Upon further inspection, this appeared to have an effect on the results making them questionable. That Level I trial would have a lesser overall quality of evidence than a Level I trial with randomization identified as a major limitation and *no effect* on the results noted.

Summary

Categorizing quality of the evidence is necessary to determine the strength of recommendation that can be made based on that evidence. The quality of evidence equation is a combination of both specific study design characteristics and key study attributes. Levels of evidence are determined based on key study design characteristics such as intervention/observation, controlled/non-controlled, randomized/non-randomized, and whether power is set and met by enrolling the required number of subjects.

The better study design provides a higher quality and reliability of evidence (higher level of evidence), making a stronger recommendation possible. Level I evidence has the highest quality and reliability of evidence. The progression from Level I to Level V evidence represents a decrease in the quality and reliability of the evidence, and consequently a lower strength of recommendation being developed. Add to this the presence or absence of key study attributes, and then the overall quality of the evidence can be determined. From this overall quality of evidence rating, a final recommendation is developed based on the available evidence.

References

1. Guyatt GH, Sackett DL, Sinclair JC, et al. Users' guides to the medical literature. IX. A method for grading health care recommendations. Evidence-Based Medicine Working Group [published erratum appears in *JAMA* 1996; 275(16):1232]. *JAMA*. 1995; 274:1800–1804.

2. McGovern DPB, Summerskill WSM, Valori RM, et al. *Key Topics in Evidence-Based Medicine*. Oxford, UK: BIOS Scientific Publishers Limited; 2001.

3. Heneghan C, Badenoch D. *Evidence-based Medicine Toolkit*. Oxford, UK: Blackwell Publishing Limited; 2006.

4. Mayer D. *Essential Evidence-Based Medicine*. Cambridge, UK: Cambridge University Press; 2004.

5. U.S. Preventive Services Task Force. *Guide to Clinical Preventive Services*. 2nd ed. Baltimore, MD: Williams & Wilkins; 1996.

6. The Canadian Task Force on the Periodic Health Examination. *The Canadian Guide to Clinical Preventive Health Care*. Ottawa: Health Canada; 1994.

7. Cook DJ, Guyatt GH, Laupacis A, et al. Rules of evidence and clinical recommendations on the use of antithrombotic agents. *Chest*. 1992; 102(4 suppl):305S–311S.

8. Sackett DL. Rules of evidence and clinical recommendations. *Can J Cardiol*. 1993; 9:487–489.

9. Guyatt G, Rennie D, eds. *User's Guides to the Medical Literature*. Chicago, IL: AMA Press; 2002.

10. Cook DJ, Guyatt GH, Laupacis A, et al. Rules of evidence and clinical recommendations on the use of antithrombotic agents. *Chest*. 1992; 102(4 suppl):305S–311S.

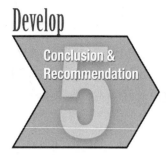

Develop

Conclusion &
Recommendation

5

Chapter 7

Develop a Conclusion and Recommendation

Patrick J. Bryant

Step 5 – Develop a Conclusion and Recommendation

The fifth step of the 5-Step Evidence-Based Medicine Process, Develop a Conclusion and Recommendation, may be the most important task and yet can be the most challenging for the practitioner. This is the step that provides a solid and defendable recommendation. The degree of confidence in the recommendation and the justifications supporting that recommendation are based on the quality of evidence available. Essentially, the recommendation is as strong as the supporting evidence. A recommendation developed following the 5-Step Evidence-Based Medicine Process is easy to support and defend because the highest quality of evidence has been utilized.

A recommendation developed following the 5-Step Evidence-Based Medicine Process is easy to support and defend when necessary. Essentially, the recommendation is as strong as the supporting evidence.

Organizing the Pertinent Information

Once the evidence has been retrieved, analyzed, and categorized by quality, sorting the pertinent information by level of evidence is extremely helpful to begin developing a conclusion. By organizing the evidence from the highest to lowest in confidence (levels of evidence and major limitations), the practitioner can begin to identify the most reliable information to develop a conclusion (see **Figure 7.1**).

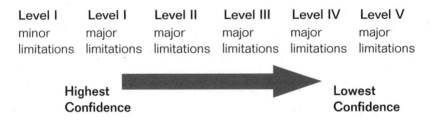

| Level I | Level I | Level II | Level III | Level IV | Level V |
| minor limitations | major limitations | major limitations | major limitations | major limitations | major limitations |

Highest Confidence   **Lowest Confidence**

Figure 7.1: Sort Pertinent Studies by Level of Evidence and Major Limitations

Organizing pertinent information by level of evidence and using a tool called Summary Table of Evidence Evaluated brings clarity to what the evidence is supporting.

The studies with the highest confidence can be organized even further using the Summary Table of Evidence Evaluated (see table in **Figure 7.2** and also the "EBM Tool Kit" at the end of this book). This table summarizes not only the level of evidence, but also the study outcome and major limitations from the Ten Major Considerations identified in Step 3: Evaluate Literature. Clar-

Clinical Question - Is Drug A as efficacious and safe as Drug B, currently on formulary?

Article	Outcome	Level of Evidence	Major Limitations
Study #1	Equivalent	I	No Major
Study #2	Equivalent	II	Major-power
Study #3	Equivalent	II	Major-power

Figure 7.2: Summary Table of Evidence Evaluated

ity emerges by observing all the evidence presented in the same table at the same time.

Developing a Conclusion from the Summary

The conclusion becomes more apparent as results from the highest level of evidence are compared and contrasted in the Summary Table of Evidence Evaluated. By reviewing these findings in more detail, the practitioner will be able to identify the differences between the highest quality trials. These differences are important in fine-tuning the conclusion and one's degree of confidence in that conclusion.

Example 7.1. Developing a Conclusion

Clinical Question - Is Drug A as efficacious and safe as Drug B, currently on formulary?

Summary Table of Evidence Evaluated

Article	Outcome	Level of Evidence	Major Limitations
Study #1	Equivalent	I	No Major
Study #2	Equivalent	II	Major-power
Study #3	Equivalent	II	Major-power and dose for Drug A

For example, a conclusion that Drug A has equivalent efficacy compared to Drug B can be made from the single Level I trial with no major limitations. The major limitation of power not being met puts the first Level II trial in question. When power has not been met and there is no difference between treatment groups, the concern is that a difference may have been shown if enough patients had been entered to meet power (see Chapter 2: Basics for Interpretation).

After careful review, it is determined that there is no way to assess whether this major limitation had an effect on the overall study results; however, one should assume that it *did* affect the overall results. The second Level II trial has this same major limitation in addition to a question about whether the higher dose used for Drug A may have given that drug an unfair advantage. If a normal therapeutic dose of Drug A would have been used, Drug A may have been less effective than Drug B. There is no way to determine if this major limitation had an effect on the overall study results. To be on the conservative side, one should assume that this major limitation *did* have an effect on the overall results.

This example illustrates the necessity for including the major limitations to help determine overall confidence in a study's results. If major limitations are not taken into consideration, an inappropriate conclusion may be reached. Even with a high level of evidence, overall reliability of the trial could be reduced by one major limitation such as dissimilar groups after randomization. (For a list of the Ten Major Considerations, see Chapter 5: Evaluate Literature.)

Key Idea

Incorporating the identified major limitations assists in determining overall reliability of the evidence.

It is crucial to determine whether the results appear to be affected by an identified major limitation. After this determination, a decision can be made to either include the trial results as reliable or discredit findings and exclude the trial. For instance, in Example 7.1, if Study #1 had dissimilarity in demographics between treatment groups (e.g., height of the patients), this has nothing to do with efficacy outcomes in this case. It would be appropriate to conclude that Drug A and Drug B are equivalent regarding efficacy. This case illustrates the importance of determining the impact each identified major limitation could have on overall study results.

Developing a Recommendation from the Conclusion

From Conclusion to Recommendation

Even the simplest decision involves a process that must occur between forming a conclusion and developing a recommendation. Three components are involved in this process (see **Figure 7.3**).

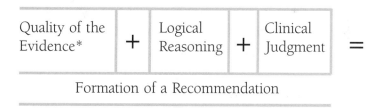

| Quality of the Evidence* | + | Logical Reasoning | + | Clinical Judgment | = |

Formation of a Recommendation

*Quality of the evidence, major strengths, and any major limitations are considerations.

Figure 7.3: Components Required to Develop a Recommendation

The first component (quality of the evidence) is a result of Step 3: Evaluate Literature and Step 4: Categorize the Quality of Evidence of the 5-Step Evidence-Based Medicine Process outlined in this book. The quality of the available evidence is considered in addition to major strengths and limitations of studies that make up this available evidence. When developing a recommendation, the practitioner should know that the overall reliability of the evidence is important.

Logical reasoning, the second component, requires both deductive and inductive reasoning. This component provides practicality in forming the recommendation. For instance, when no head-to-head comparative trials exist for two drugs, other trials with identical control groups for each drug in similar patient populations may be used along with logical reasoning to draw conclusions that go into the recommendation.

The third component, clinical judgment, comes from experience as a clinical practitioner. Clinical judgment fills in gaps where evidence does not exist or is weak. For instance, a practitioner's clinical experience reveals that with a specific patient, drugs from the same pharmacological class have different degrees of efficacy. Based on this clinical judgment, the practitioner may suggest changing to a different drug in the same pharmacological class to assist in identifying the optimal agent.

Key Idea

Conclusions drawn from the evidence analyzed assist in the development of recommendation statements. Reliability of the evidence combined with logical reasoning and clinical judgment all factor into the clinical decision making process.

For extremely complex decisions leading to recommendations, formal decision analysis processes are used.[1-4] The primary tool utilized is the decision tree. Discussion on the use of decision trees and formal decision analysis processes are beyond the scope of this book. A detailed tutorial on performing this type of analysis is available.[5]

Type of Decision

Two types of clinical decisions will be discussed in this book—individual patient and population-based. An individual patient decision is represented by a typical treatment plan developed for a single patient. A population-based decision is represented by a formulary management clinical decision (see table in **Figure 7.4**, page 111). Both decisions are important and will affect health care for patients.

The population-based decision is typically made in a more conservative manner since many patients will be affected and little is known about the specifics of each patient in this population. When details about a single patient's disease and medication history are known, the practitioner can customize the decision to fit that individual patient. Knowing these specifics allows the practitioner to use clinical judgment associated with that individual. With an understanding of the type of clinical decision being made (individual patient versus population-based), the practitioner can modify the final recommendation to fit the type of decision.

Key Idea

Population-based decisions require a more conservative approach since specifics about the individual patients that will be affected are unknown.

Example 7.2. Developing a Recommendation Based on Type of Decision

Clinical Question – Is Drug A as efficacious and safe as Drug B, currently on the formulary?

Here is what we know from the evidence:

1. Conclusion from evidence – Drug A and Drug B have equivalent efficacy and safety with no specific advantage of one over the other. Drug A is considerably more expensive than Drug B.

2. This is supported by a Level I trial with no major limitations.

3. The two Level II trials are not considered since

they were not powered to show a difference, if one existed and no difference between treatment groups was noted.

4. This is a population-based decision; therefore, a conservative stance needs to be taken with the clinical decision to be made here. If this were an individual patient decision, the practitioner would want to assess any subgroup analyses that may pertain to the specific patient. With this in mind, a completely different recommendation could be required.

Recommendation Statement: I do not recommend adding Drug A to the formulary. (Note: The degree of confidence one has in this recommnedation still needs to be fully determined to adjust the overall tone of the statement. This will be explained in the next section.)

Confidence of the Recommendation

The confidence of a recommendation depends on the quality of evidence supporting that recommendation statement. The degree of confidence one has in the evidence is important when determining how strongly to state the recommendation. To assist in determining strength of the recommendation statement, the Grade of Recommendation Tool is used. The highest level of evidence (Level I) is also the evidence that carries the greatest confidence (see **Figure 7.5**, page 112, and also the "EBM Tool Kit" at the end of this book). For instance, a Grade A Recommendation would be based on Level I evidence. Unless major limitations exist that would cause concern with the study's integrity, this grade allows a strong and firm recommendation statement.

Key Idea

The Grade of Recommendation Tool helps establish the firmness of the language used in the recommendation statement.

Type of Clinical Decision	Manner in Which Decision Is Made	
	Less Conservative	*More Conservative*
Individual Patient Decision	• Only one patient involved. • The patient's medical history and background are known in addition to drug allergies. • Specific co-morbid disease states such as liver and/or kidney impairment are known. • Prognosis is known for this specific patient. • Also known is whether the drug in question is the last option to treat the disease for this patient.	
Population-Based Decision		• Potentially, a large number of patients will be affected. • Individual patient medical history and background are not known, including drug allergies. • Specific co-morbid disease states are unknown. • Prognosis of each patient in the population is not known. • Also not known is whether the drug in question is the last treatment option for each patient.

Figure 7.4: Individual Patient versus Population-Based Decisions

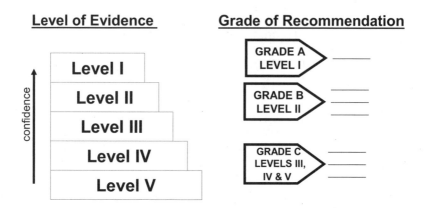

Figure 7.5: Correlation among Confidence in Evidence, Level of Evidence, and Grade of Recommendation

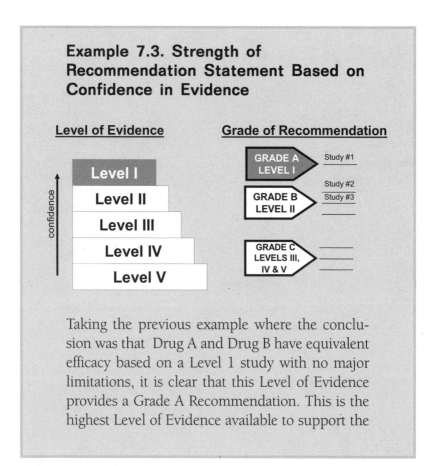

Example 7.3. Strength of Recommendation Statement Based on Confidence in Evidence

Taking the previous example where the conclusion was that Drug A and Drug B have equivalent efficacy based on a Level 1 study with no major limitations, it is clear that this Level of Evidence provides a Grade A Recommendation. This is the highest Level of Evidence available to support the recommendation and, therefore, a strong and firm tone should be used in the recommendation statement if no major limitations exist.

Knowing that a Grade A Recommendation designation allows the highest degree of firmness in the language used to develop the recommendation statement, a firm recommendation statement can now be developed for this situation. For instance, I strongly recommend to not add Drug A to the formulary.

Format for the Recommendation

Recommendations should include a statement with justification points that support the recommendation (see **Figure 7.6** and also the "EBM Tool Kit" at the end of this book). Although various formats can be used to present a recommendation, a clear and concise statement is important to ensure effective communication. This template can be modified to fit various styles, but two primary components should be present—a clear and concise recommendation statement followed by supportive justification points.

THE RECOMMENDATION STATEMENT

JUSTIFICATION IN A BULLET FORMAT
- Efficacy
- Safety
- Other special considerations/populations
- Cost

Figure 7.6: Format for a Recommendation

Example 7.4. The Recommendation Statement

I strongly recommend that Drug A not replace Drug B on the formulary, but be reserved as second-line therapy for allergic conjunctivitis only after Drug B has been tried and failed.

Support for the Recommendation

Justification points provide clear and concise support, similar to "pillars," for the recommendation statement (see **Figure 7.7**). Each justification point includes the efficacy, safety, special considerations/special populations, and cost associated with a specific situation. Information obtained from the evidence should be addressed under each of these considerations:

Efficacy

❏ Summary of the highest level of evidence trial(s) being used to develop the recommendation statement.

❏ Specifically what that evidence confirms. Any major limitations identified along with the determined impact that those limitations may have on the results, especially the primary outcome measure(s).

❏ Any outcomes that are of interest to the clinical question.

Safety

❏ Description of adverse drug reactions noted especially those different from the comparison group(s).

❏ A statement of overall safety profile and any safety concern(s). This should be obtained from information that includes the greatest number of patients exposed (usually, the Package Insert/Prescribing Information) to attempt to identify rare adverse drug reactions.

Special considerations/special populations

❏ This is a very broad scope category, and the content is

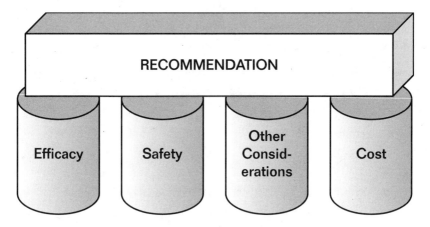

Figure 7.7: Justification Points Support the Recommendation

highly dependent upon the defined clinical question. Some types of special considerations that would be appropriate to include are differences in dosing convenience and route of administration between the drugs in question.

❑ Any knowledge gained that addresses the advantages and/ or disadvantages of the study drug over existing therapy.

❑ Specific populations that need to be highlighted due to the drug's benefit or disadvantages on those populations should be addressed.

❑ Any knowledge gained from the study that provides an understanding of how and where this drug fits in overall therapeutic strategies and standard practice guidelines should be included.

Cost

❑ Differences in cost between the treatments studied including nursing/pharmacy and other related costs, if possible.

❑ Differences in cost compared to current standard of care treatment.

❑ Any impact associated with these differences in cost (both savings and/or expenditures).

The following example illustrates effective use of justification points to support/defend the previously developed recommendation statement.

Example 7.5. Justification for the Recommendation

I recommend that Drug A not replace Drug B on the formulary, but be reserved as second-line therapy for allergic conjunctivitis only after Drug B has been tried and failed. The following reasons support this recommendation:

Efficacy	One Level I trial with no major limitations confirms that Drug A and Drug B are equivalent in efficacy.
	Two additional Level II trials supported the above finding. Major limitations that make these results less reliable include 1) no power calculation for either trial and 2) in one trial higher than FDA-recommended doses of Drug B were used.
Safety	Safety results from this trial are similar to the Prescribing Information available for each drug and confirms that the safety profiles are similar for both drugs with the exception that Drug A has a higher incidence of burning and stinging of the eyes.
Special Considerations/ Special Populations	No special considerations have been identified. There are no special population issues identified.
Cost	Cost for Drug A is considerably higher than for Drug B since Drug B has a generic equivalent.

Note: Level of Evidence is a way to communicate with other individuals who know this 5-Step Evidence-Based Medicine Process; however, be prepared to describe each level in a manner that others who are *not* familiar with this method to categorize quality can understand. For instance, in Example 7.5, the efficacy justification section could be rewritten in more generic terms such as, "One high quality, randomized controlled trial meeting power with no major limitations confirms that Drug A and Drug B are equivalent in efficacy."

Summary

Developing a conclusion and recommendation can be challenging, but the result is a reproducible and defendable recommendation when it is done based on evidence. Utilizing the Summary Table of Evidence Evaluated tool, the pertinent information can be organized in a manner so that a clear conclusion becomes apparent. Knowing the type of decision being made will help to determine if the recommendation must remain conservative. A more conservative recommendation should be developed for population-based decisions since there are considerably fewer specifics known in this situation than with an individual patient decision. The level of evidence and presence of major limitations will assist in determining the confidence one can place in the recommendation.

Three separate components are involved when developing a recommendation statement: quality of the evidence, logical reasoning, and clinical judgment. The recommendation statement should be supported by justification points addressing efficacy, safety, special considerations/special populations, and cost. Essentially, the recommendation is as strong as the supporting evidence. Using the 5-Step Evidence-Based Medicine Process described in this book provides a recommendation that is easy to support and defend.

References

1. Gross R, ed. *Decisions and Evidence in Medical Practice: Applying Evidence-Based Medicine to Clinical Decision Making*. St. Louis, MO: Mosby; 2001.

2. Mayer D, ed. *Essential Evidence-Based Medicine*. New York, NY: Cambridge University Press; 2004.

3. Jenicek M. *Foundations of Evidence-Based Medicine*. New York, NY: The Parthenon Publishing Group Inc.; 2003.

4. Sarnes M. Making a Pharmacotherapy Decision Using a Decision–Analytic Framework. In: Chiquette E, Posey LM, eds. *Evidence-Based Pharmacotherapy*. Washington, D.C.: American Pharmacists Association; 2007.

5. Detsky AS, Naglie G, Krahn MD, et.al. Primer on medical decision analysis: Part 1—getting started. *Med Decision Making*. 1997; 17(2):123–125.

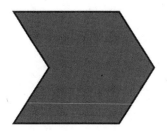

Chapter 8

Alternative Sources of Evidence

Heather A. Pace

Alternative Sources of Evidence

This chapter presents alternative sources of evidence used for clinical decision making and outlines the strengths and weaknesses of each. Systematic reviews, meta-analyses, narrative reviews, and practice guidelines are useful tools, but without applying the process of evidence-based medicine they can lead to inappropriate and possibly dangerous clinical decisions.

Systematic Reviews and Meta-Analyses

Systematic reviews and meta-analyses are methods used to summarize large numbers of clinical trials and, if used carefully, can be valuable tools for the busy practitioner. The general process for systematic reviews and meta-analyses is similar. Both methods evaluate and combine results from a compilation of randomized controlled trials pertaining to the specific clinical question at hand. The key difference between these two methods is in the outcome and how each reaches its conclusion. Meta-analyses employ statistical methods to combine results of primary trials and produce a single pooled estimate of an intervention's effect.

Meta-analyses establish criteria to ensure that the data from single trials are homogenous to allow for the creation of new data from statistical analysis, whereas systematic reviews do not produce new data, merely a combination of the existing data from the single trials. It is important to consider the quality of the new data produced by a meta-analysis as this can affect the overall reliability of the meta-analysis results. Systematic reviews do not employ statistical methods and produce qualitative results rather than quantitative results. Both methods can produce strong evidence or potentially poor quality evidence; therefore, caution is advised and some form of critical evaluation is required to determine the quality of this evidence.

Systematic reviews and meta-analyses can be useful in the following cases:

- ❑ When primary data is conflicting or in disagreement as to the direction or magnitude of effect
- ❑ If sample sizes in primary research are too small to detect an effect
- ❑ If large trials simply are not feasible

Example 8.1. Using Multiple Studies

"Does estrogen replacement therapy increase the risk of breast cancer?" Because the incidence of breast cancer is so low, it may not occur often enough to answer the question based on individual studies. Combining multiple studies may provide sufficient incidence to answer the question.

Oftentimes meta-analyses can provide conclusions about a treatment effect that cannot be drawn from individual trials and may possibly answer questions not addressed in single trials. The purpose of conducting a meta-analysis is to:

- ❑ Increase statistical power, resolve uncertainty when single trials disagree

- ❑ Improve estimates of size effect
- ❑ Answer new questions (use the old data in a new way)
- ❑ Bring about improvements in quality of research

Key Idea

Meta-analyses employ statistical methods to combine results of primary trials and produce a single pooled quantitative estimate of an intervention's effect (new data produced), while systematic reviews produce non-statistical, qualitative results (no new data produced).

Systematic reviews and meta-analyses can be described as scientific investigations with predefined methods and original studies as the subjects.[1] As mentioned earlier, quality needs to be analyzed just as with single trials. The methods to determine the quality of systematic reviews and meta-analyses are similar to those used for individual clinical trials and are described in Chapter 5: Step 3–Evaluate Literature. Similar considerations as those used for clinical trials are examined to determine the quality of the resulting evidence provided by systematic reviews and meta-analyses. Certain design characteristics that should be evaluated include the following[2]:

- ❑ Is there a clear objective stated?
- ❑ Was a comprehensive search used to identify all relevant studies? (recruitment methods)
- ❑ Are the inclusion/exclusion criteria for the selection of studies appropriate?
- ❑ Are the individual studies evaluated for validity and quality?
- ❑ Are the individual study characteristics described?
- ❑ Is there an appropriate quantitative data synthesis? (appropriate statistical analysis)
- ❑ Are both clinical and statistical significance reported?
- ❑ Are the results generalizable to clinical practice?

While systematic reviews and meta-analyses can offer advantages over single studies, they are not as useful for patient-specific questions. Because of the potential in design flaws, introduction of bias, or overall false conclusions, results from systematic reviews and meta-analyses should be applied with caution and should not be the sole source of evidence when making a clinical decision.

Narrative Reviews

Narrative or non-systematic reviews lack an orderly method for identifying and analyzing data. The biggest difference between narrative reviews and systematic reviews or meta-analysis is that narrative reviews do not provide pooled results from primary trials. Narrative reviews often provide a broad overview of a specific topic, including disease pathology, diagnosis, prevention, and multiple therapeutic interventions. Conclusions can be less evidence-based and affected by the opinions of the authors. Oftentimes considered a tertiary source of literature, narrative reviews are useful in establishing background information but should not be used as supporting evidence for a recommendation. Moreover, narrative reviews often contain extensive bibliographies and can provide an excellent source for identifying literature surrounding a specific subject. The table in **Figure 8.1** provides an overview of systematic reviews, meta-analysis, and narrative reviews.

Practice Guidelines

A lack of understanding about the requirements for guideline development could lead to either inappropriate interpretation or acceptance of inappropriate enforcement levels of biased guideline recommendations.[2]

Feature	Narrative Review	Systematic Review	Meta Analysis
Clinical question	Often broadly defined	Clearly defined and focused	Clearly defined and focused
Literature search	Methods not usually explicitly described	Predefined strategy, explicit and comprehensive	Predefined strategy, explicit and comprehensive
Studies included	Inclusion methods not usually described	Predefined inclusion and exclusion criteria	Predefined inclusion and exclusion criteria
Unpublished literature included	Not usually	Possibly	Possibly
Blinding of reviewers	No	Yes	Yes
Analysis of data	Variable and subjective	Rigorous and objective—no new data produced	Rigorous and objective—new data produced
Results statistically evaluated	No	No	Yes
Type of results	Qualitative	Qualitative	Quantitative

Adapted from Pinsky L, Deyo R. Clinical guidelines: a strategy for translating evidence into practice. In: Geyman J, Deyo R, Ramsey S, eds. *Evidence Based Clinical Practice*. 1st ed. Woburn, MA: Butterworth-Heinemann; 2000:119–123.

Figure 8.1: Comparisons of Characteristics of Reviews

Practice guidelines help to provide consistent health care, establish practice standards, and aid in guiding clinical decisions. Practice guidelines can be flawed, making it important to evaluate and apply certain evidence-based medicine principles. The information used to support and develop the guidelines should be evaluated as well as the overall quality of the guideline.

The first consideration when evaluating a guideline is to determine the method used to develop it. Not all practice guidelines are evidence-based; however, many guidelines are moving towards an evidence-based process. The reasons for this shift include a rapid increase of available information, greater availability of treatments, an increase in the number of technologies of unproven efficacy, and wide variations in practice habits among physicians.[3]

Guidelines can be evidence- or consensus-based. Evidence-based guidelines follow a rigorous process to identify and evaluate literature for developing recommendations, whereas a consensus process relies on the experience of experts to develop and support recommendations. ATP III (Adult Treatment Panel III) and JNC7 (the Seventh Report of the Joint National Committee on Prevention, Detection, Evaluation, and Treatment of High Blood Pressure) are examples of some of the most widely used evidence-based guidelines.

Although an evidence-based development process is preferred, consensus can be useful in situations where limited evidence or information exists. In these cases, guidelines can help establish practice standards. Guidelines can be a hybrid of the two methods, combining both evidence-based and expert opinions. This approach can be useful when practice trends are needed to fill-in "gaps" left by poor evidence or lack of evidence. The table in **Figure 8.2** represents the differences between the two types of guidelines.

Evidence-Based Guidelines	Consensus Guidelines
Principles of evidence-based medicine	Principles of clinical observation
Reasoning based on clinical studies	Reasoning based on pathophysiology
Guidelines based on evaluation of medical literature	Guidelines based on expert opinion

Figure 8.2: Differences Between Evidence-Based and Consensus Guidelines

Credentials of the authors and the source of the document are important areas to consider when evaluating the quality of practice guidelines. Ideally authors or an organization are experts in the specific field. For instance, the American Diabetes Association and the American College of Obstetricians and Gynecologists are considered examples of reputable organizations and should be expected to produce reliable, accurate guidelines; however, one should still determine the method used to develop the guideline: evidence-based, consensus-based, or hybrid.

Practice guidelines should also be periodically updated to keep up with changing practice, new treatments, and recent evidence. The incorporation of new data in updates strengthens the recommendation and value of the guideline. It is important to verify the date of development of a guideline to ensure recommendations are based on the most recent evidence and treatments available.

When evaluating practice guidelines, consider the following questions:

❑ Development method of guideline (consensus versus evidence-based)?

❑ Are the recommendations valid and reliable?

❑ Are the recommendations generalizable?

❑ Was there a peer review process?

❑ Were literature search methods outlined and explained?

❑ Are the guidelines reviewed and updated on a regular basis?

Summary

The evidence-based medicine process is not only useful and important in evaluating single randomized controlled trials, but it is also helpful to determine the quality and reliability of alternative sources of evidence used for clinical decision making. The application of this process will ensure that information is used appropriately to support clinical decisions and recommendations. Without the use of this process, systematic reviews, meta-analyses, narrative reviews, and practice guidelines could potentially lead to inappropriate and dangerous clinical decisions.

References

1. Cook DJ, Mulrow CD, Haynes RB. Systematic reviews: synthesis of best evidence for clinical decisions. *Ann Intern Med.* 1997; 126:376–380.

2. Moores K. Evidence-Based Clinical Practice Guidelines. In: Malone P, Kier K, Stanovich J. *Drug Information: A Guide for Pharmacists.* 3rd ed. McGraw Hill; 2006:289–338.

3. Lewis TA, Fineberg HV, Mosteller F. Findings for public health from meta-analysis. *Ann Review of Public Health.* May 1985; 6:1–20.

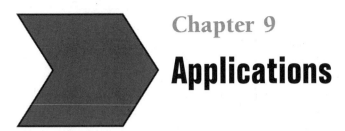

Chapter 9

Applications

Lindsey N. Schnabel & Heather A. Pace

Applications

Incorporating Evidence-Based Clinical Decision Making into Clinical Practice

How do practitioners incorporate evidence-based decision making into clinical practice? By following the five-step process outlined throughout this book, pharmacy practitioners can assess the evidence available and make either 1) *firm* recommendations and decisions based on results of rigorously controlled investigations or 2) *cautious* recommendations and decisions when results of uncontrolled clinical observations exist **(Figure 9.1)**. Evidence-based medicine, when used in pharmacy, is applied in various situations. This chapter will examine several examples of how pharmacy practitioners can use evidence-based medicine in clinical practice when making both individual patient decisions as well as population-based decisions.

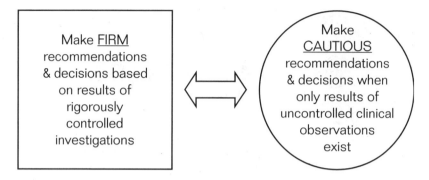

Figure 9.1: Explanation of Differences in *Firm* and *Cautious* Recommendations Based on Trial Type

Individual patient decisions

Individual patient recommendations differ from population-based decisions in that individual patient decisions require a less conservative approach.

Individual patient decisions are made frequently in pharmacy and often require a *less* conservative approach due to the fact that more information is available regarding an individual versus an entire population. Practitioners must look at the patient as a whole and consider many factors when making a recommendation or decision regarding an individual's health. As discussed previously, it is imperative to consider efficacy, safety, special considerations/special populations, and cost when making a clinical decision or recommendation. This also applies to individual patients.

The clinician should apply the 5-Step Evidence-Based Medicine Process to determine if the treatment option is efficacious. Various sources of evidence should be reviewed such as interventional or observational clinical trials, case control studies, case series, or individual case studies. By assessing risk versus benefit, the practitioner can determine if the efficacy of the therapy outweighs the harm if any it may cause to the patient.

Other important aspects to consider when looking at the safety justification of a patient-specific decision are allergies, concomitant medications and potential drug interactions, current disease states and interactions that may be associated with them, and compliance/adherence concerns.

Special populations that should be considered include dosing convenience, route of administration, specific situations that may affect the patient positively or negatively, and advantages or disadvantages over lack of treatment or existing treatment. Specifically, "Is there a population that may especially benefit from the recommendation?" An angiotensin-converting enzyme inhibitor, for instance, would benefit a kidney failure patient who also has hypertension.

Finally, cost should be considered. "Can the patient afford the treatment?" "Are there patient assistance programs available to help with affordability of the therapy?" "Is there a significant cost associated with the treatment such as travel expenses or medical devices used for administration?" "Would any additional cost be outweighed by preventing future complications or morbidity or mortality?"

By factoring efficacy, safety, special considerations/special populations, and cost into forming a decision as well as assessing risk versus benefit, practitioners can be assured that an appropriate individual patient decision is made. Chapter 7: Step 5 – Develop a Conclusion and Recommendation provides additional factors to consider for each of these catagories.

Population-based decisions

Key Idea

Population-based recommendations differ from individual patient recommendations in that population decisions require a more conservative approach.

Population-based clinical decisions differ from individual ones in that a *more* conservative approach is required because fewer specifics are known. When formulating a recommendation for a population such as a medication class review, comparative analyses, or a formulary request, the clinician's decision is affecting a large number of people who have many different disease states, different medication regimens, and different compliance issues. These decisions, similar to individual patient decisions, also require the practitioner to consider efficacy, safety, special considerations/special populations, and cost when making a recommendation.

The efficacy justification to support population-based decisions often is derived from evidence such as interventional or observational clinical trials, case control studies, or well designed meta-analyses or systematic reviews. The safety considerations of a population-based decision should be assessed by reviewing the evidence as well as the most current prescribing information.

As with individual clinical decisions, it is imperative that the following special considerations/special populations are taken into account for population-based recommendations: dosing convenience, route of administration, specific situations that may affect the population positively or negatively, and advantages or disadvantages of the treatment.

When formulating a recommendation for a population, practitioners have fewer known specifics regarding prescription coverage, patient income, and other variables; therefore, cost is typically one of the final components to consider. Sometimes the question is asked, "How much better should one drug be in terms of efficacy, safety, or special considerations/special populations to justify the additional expense?" If efficacy, safety, and special considerations/special populations are the same between comparative drugs, one can consider cost to be the primary determinant. Chapter 7: Step 5 – Develop a Conclusion and Recommendation provides additional factors to consider for each of these catagories.

Examples

The following examples are provided to illustrate application of the evidence-based process described in this book to both individual patient and population-based decisions.

Example 9.1. Individual Patient Clinical Decision/Recommendation

This example illustrates how to use the 5-Step Evidence-Based Medicine Process to assist in making a clinical decision/recommendation for an individual patient.

A physician wants to give BP, a male patient, Drug A for treatment of his osteoporosis instead of Drug B because Drug A can be given once per month whereas Drug B requires weekly administration. Somewhere the pharmacist read or heard that Drug A was not as effective in male osteoporosis as Drug B. Before the pharmacist calls the physician to discuss this issue, he or she should conduct an evidence-based medicine analysis to confirm that Drug A is not as effective as Drug B in male osteoporosis.

Patient Background:

   63-year-old male

   No known drug allergies

Past medical history:

   Hypertension—controlled on lisinopril

   Type 2 diabetes—controlled on metformin and insulin glargine

   Hypercholesterolemia—uncontrolled on simvastatin; ezetimibe added at most recent visit with physician

Prescription coverage that discounts all medications

Step 1: Define the Clinical Question

❑ Determine the actual question being asked so that an appropriate response is formed. For this example, the question would be "Is Drug A as effective as Drug B in the treatment of male osteoporosis for BP?"

Step 2: Retrieve Pertinent Information

A literature search was performed using two databases and the following search terms: Drug A (brand and generic names), Drug B (brand and generic names), osteoporosis, male. After reviewing the search results from both databases using appropriate limits and the search and sift technique, the clinician found two key articles. The clinician performed a bibliographic search by reviewing the references of the two articles found. This technique led to a case series. Overall, the literature search revealed the following articles:

❑ Article #1 – A randomized, double-blind, parallel group study in male patients with osteoporosis compared Drugs A and B. Power was set and met; that is, sample size was adequate to show a difference between study groups, if a difference really exists. One major limitation was noted; the groups were not similar after randomization. No other limitations were identified from the ten major considerations list. The results of the study showed that Drug B was superior to Drug A for the treatment of male osteoporosis, and this difference was statistically significant (p=0.001). There was no difference in the incidence or severity of adverse drug reactions between the two drugs. No special considerations/special populations were noted.

❏ Article #2 – A randomized, double-blind, crossover study in male patients with osteoporosis compared Drugs A and B for treatment. Power was set and met, thus indicating an adequate sample size has been used to show a difference between Drugs A and B, if a difference really exists. No other major limitations were noted. The results of this study showed that Drugs A and B are equivalent in efficacy for the treatment of male osteoporosis ($p=0.26$). In addition, no difference in the incidence or severity of adverse drug reactions between the two drugs was noted. No special considerations/special populations were identified. The two drugs were similar in price.

❏ Article #3 – A case series of male patients with osteoporosis were studied. These patients were observed over a 1-year period after being placed on Drug A by the primary physician. There was an improvement noted in bone density tests after 1 year of receiving Drug A. Some adverse drug reactions were noted, but they were anticipated based on the package insert information and were not severe. No special considerations/special populations were noted.

❏ The two drugs are similar in price; however, Drug A is covered by prescription insurance.

Step 3: Evaluate Literature
❏ Efficacy
  • Critically evaluate each trial and determine if the article supports or refutes the use of Drug A over Drug B.

- Article #1 – The results of the study showed that Drug B was superior to Drug A for the treatment of male osteoporosis, and this difference was statistically significant (p=0.001).

- Article #2 – The results of this study showed that Drugs A and B are equivalent in efficacy for the treatment of male osteoporosis (p=0.26).

- Article #3 – There was an improvement noted in bone density tests after 1 year of receiving Drug A; however, statistics were not performed since there was no comparison group.

- Establish if each trial has major or minor limitations.

    - Article #1 – The groups were not similar in baseline bone mineral density scores after randomization, and this appeared to have potentially affected the results. No other major limitations were identified.

    - Article #2 – No major limitations from the ten major considerations list were noted.

    - Article #3 – This study was a case series and, therefore, did not have a comparative group. Due to this study design, several of the ten major considerations were considered to be major limitations.

❑ Safety

- Assess risk versus benefit of Drug A versus Drug B versus no treatment.

- Article #1 – No difference was noted in the incidence or severity of adverse drug reactions between the two drugs.

- Article #2 – No difference was noted in the incidence or severity of adverse drug reactions between the two drugs.

- Article #3 – Some adverse drug reactions were noted, but they were anticipated based on the package insert information for Drug A and were not severe. Note there was no comparison group.

❑ Special considerations/special populations

• Establish if Drug A is dosed more or less conveniently than Drug B.

- Drug A is dosed once monthly compared to Drug B, which is weekly.

• Does the route of administration vary between drugs?

• Determine any potential advantages or disadvantages of Drug A versus Drug B.

Step 4: Categorize the Quality of Evidence

❑ Determine the level of evidence for each trial, including the major and minor limitations identified.

• Article #1 is a Level I trial with the major limitation that the two groups are not similar after randomization, which appears to have affected the results.

• Article #2 is a Level I trial with minor limitations.

• Article #3 is a Level V trial with major limitations.

Article	Support/Refute	Level of Evidence	Major/Minor Limitations
1	S	I	Major-Randomization that discredited the results
2	S	I	Minor
3	S	V	Major

Figure 9.2: Summary Table of Evidence Evaluated for Example 9.1 – Individual Patient Decision

Step 5: Develop a Conclusion and Recommendation

❏ Develop a conclusion regarding the overall *efficacy* based on the evidence.

• Drug A is equivalent to Drug B in overall efficacy.

❏ Develop a conclusion regarding the overall *safety* based on the evidence.

• Drugs A and B have similar safety profiles.

❏ Review patient's allergies and potential drug–drug or drug–disease interactions to limit adverse events.

• No drug–drug interactions were identified with current therapy.

❏ Develop a conclusion regarding any special considerations/special populations.

• Drug A is administered significantly less frequently than Drug B.

❏ Develop a conclusion regarding the overall cost of medication specific to this individual patient based on the following:

- Can the patient afford this medication?
  - Insurance coverage

    BP's insurance covers Drug A.
  - Patient assistance programs available
- Are there other cost concerns associated with the treatment?
- Are there long-term cost-saving benefits of Drug A or Drug B?

❑ Assign the appropriate grade of recommendation based on the quality of evidence available **(Figure 9.3)**.

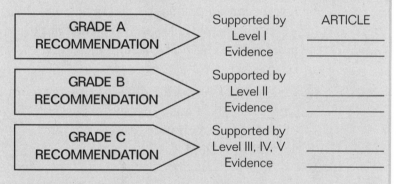

Figure 9.3: This Grade of Recommendation Table Is Used to Develop Each Grade of Recommendation by Tracking Articles and Levels of Evidence (also located in the "EBM Tool Kit")

❑ Develop a recommendation based on conclusions made and applied to this individual patient.

❑ Example:

I strongly recommend using Drug A for the treatment of osteoporosis in BP for the following reasons: (Grade A Recommendation)

- Efficacy – A Level I trial showed that Drugs A and B were equivalent in efficacy for treating male osteoporosis. A second Level

I trial showed that Drug B was superior to Drug A in the treatment of male osteoporosis; however, this trial had a major limitation that discredited the results. As additional support, a case series noted an improvement in the bone density test after 1 year of receiving Drug A.

- Safety – There appeared to be no difference in adverse drug reactions between Drugs A and B. No drug–drug interactions were noted with BP's current medication regimen. BP has no known drug allergies; therefore, it's not an issue.

- Special considerations/special populations – Drug A would allow the patient once monthly dosing, thus possibly increasing compliance.

- Cost – Drugs A and B are similar in price. Drug A will be a less expensive choice for BP since his prescription insurance coverage includes Drug A.

Example 9.2. Population-Based Decision/Recommendation

This example illustrates how to compile a class review or comparative review to assist in the formulary management decision making process.

Step 1: Define the Clinical Question

❑ Determine the actual question being asked so that an appropriate response is formed. For this example, the question would be "Is there a specific drug(s) that is superior to the others within the class?"

Step 2: Retrieve Pertinent Information

❏ Become familiar with class by reading tertiary textbook resources, compendia class summaries, recent review articles, or class reviews.

❏ Identify medications to be compared and identify FDA-approved indications.

❏ Complete a literature search for Level I or II comparative trials by searching various databases. Using the "search and sift" technique, narrow the search to randomized, controlled trials with or without power met in human subjects. In order to ensure a thorough search is accomplished, be sure to complete a bibliographic search of all relevant articles.

• The search should compare drugs in the same class, not drugs compared to other classes or the drug compared to placebo, if possible.

• If head-to-head comparison trials do not exist, then consider using placebo-controlled trials or trials comparing the class to the same drug that maybe is outside of the class.

Step 3: Evaluate Literature

❏ Efficacy

• Review each trial and determine if the article supports or refutes the use of one drug over another.

• Establish if each trial has major or minor limitations.

❏ Safety

• Assess safety of the drugs within the class when compared in the literature.

- Obtain the most recent package inserts to help determine possible safety concerns; safety information should always be derived from package inserts rather than individual trials. Larger patient population exposure and possibly longer patient exposure are found in package inserts.

❏ Special considerations/special populations

- Establish if one drug is dosed more or less conveniently than the other(s).
- Does the route of administration vary between drugs?
- Determine if there are other potential advantages or disadvantages of the drugs within the class.

❏ Cost

- Is the cost significantly lower for one drug?
- Are there long-term cost-saving benefits?
- When formulating a recommendation for a population, fewer specifics are known regarding prescription coverage, patient income, and other variables; therefore, cost is typically one of the final components to consider when forming the recommendation.
- Identify differentiating characteristics for medications within the class by indication and use to aid in formulating evidence-based conclusion.

Step 4: Categorize the Quality of Evidence

❏ Determine the level of evidence for each trial, including the major or minor limitations identified.

Step 5: Develop a Conclusion and Recommendation (see Figure 9.2)

❑ Develop a conclusion regarding the overall efficacy based on the evidence.

❑ Develop a conclusion regarding the overall safety based on the evidence.

❑ Develop a conclusion regarding any special considerations/special populations.

❑ Develop a conclusion regarding the overall cost of medication specific to this population on the following:

- Cost of Drug X versus Drug Y
- Long-term cost benefits of either drug

❑ Assign the appropriate grade of recommendation (Figure 9.3).

❑ Develop a recommendation statement based on conclusions and grade of recommendation to be applied to this population.

❑ Formulate evidence-based recommendation statement with appropriate justification:

- Efficacy
- Safety
- Special considerations/special populations
- Cost

Example 9.3. Population-Based Decision/Recommendation

This example illustrates how to compile a comparative review to assist in the formulary management decision making process.

A physician has requested the addition of Drug X to an institution's formulary to replace Drug Y for treatment of chronic obstructive pulmonary disease (COPD). The pharmacist has been asked to complete a comparative review of the two agents. In addition, an evidence-based medicine recommendation needs to be developed that the pharmacist can present and defend at the next P&T meeting for the institution.

Step 1: Define the Clinical Question

❑ Determine the actual question being asked so that an appropriate response is formed. For this example, the question would be "Should Drug X replace Drug Y for COPD on the formulary?"

Step 2: Retrieve Pertinent Information

A search of the literature revealed the following evidence:

❑ Article #1 – A randomized, placebo-controlled trial was conducted using Drug X in patients with COPD. Power was not met, thus indicating that an adequate sample size was not used to show a difference between study groups, if a difference really exists. None of the other ten major considerations were discussed. Patients receiving Drug X showed greater improvement in trough FEV_1 over placebo ($p \leq 0.01$). These same patients also showed significant improvements in other outcome measures such as peak expiratory flow rate, decreased exacerbations, and health status scores. The only adverse effect that was noted to occur more frequently in the Drug X group was dry mouth. Patients receiving Drug X who also had impaired renal function were required to have dose frequency adjustments.

❑ Article #2 – A randomized, placebo-controlled trial was conducted using Drug X in patients with COPD. Power was set but not met, thus indicating that an adequate sample size was not used to show a difference between study groups, if a difference really exists. No other major limitations were noted. The patients receiving Drug X showed greater improvement from baseline than Drug Y in both trough FEV_1 ($p \leq 0.001$) and FVC ($p \leq 0.05$) and maintained these effects throughout the study period. Patients receiving Drug X also experienced significantly greater improvement over Drug Y in peak expiratory flow rate ($p < 0.01$). More patients in the Drug X group experienced dry mouth effects than those in the Drug Y group. Due to the strict inclusion/exclusion criteria, no special considerations/special populations were identified. Drug X is more expensive than Drug Y. Patients had more difficulty using the drug dispensing device for Drug X versus Drug Y.

❑ Article #3 – A case report described 12 patients receiving Drug X who also experienced dry mouth. These patients were observed by their family physician who prescribed the drug to treat their COPD symptoms. No details were given.

Step 3: Evaluate Literature
❑ Efficacy

- Review each trial and determine if the article supports or refutes the use of Drug X over Drug Y.

  - Article #1 – The results of the study showed that Drug X was superior to placebo, improving pulmonary function in COPD patients. Specifically, patients receiving Drug X showed greater improvement in trough FEV_1 over placebo ($p \leq 0.01$). These same patients also showed significant improvements in other outcome measures such as peak expiratory flow rate, decreased exacerbations, and health status scores.

  - Article #2 – The results of the study showed that Drug X was superior to Drug Y, improving pulmonary function in COPD patients. Specifically, patients receiving Drug X showed greater improvement from baseline than Drug Y in both trough FEV_1 ($p \leq 0.001$) and FVC ($p \leq 0.05$) and maintained these effects throughout the study period. Patients receiving Drug X also experienced significantly greater improvement over Drug Y in peak expiratory flow rate ($p < 0.01$).

  - Article #3 – No details were given regarding efficacy in this case report discussing the safety of Drug X in 12 patients.

- Establish if each trial has major or minor limitations.

  - Article #1 – Power was set, but not

met. That is, an adequate sample size was not used to show a difference between study groups, if a difference really exists. However, because there was a statistically significant difference noted with the primary endpoint for Drug X compared to placebo, this is less of a concern. None of the other ten major considerations were discussed.

- Article #2 – Power was set, but not met. That is, an adequate sample size was not used to show a difference between study groups, if a difference really exists. However, because there was a statistically significant difference noted with the primary endpoint for Drug X compared to placebo, this is less of a concern. None of the other ten major limitations were identified.

- Article #3 – This was a case report, and, therefore did not have a comparative group. Due to this, there were several major limitations.

❑ Safety

• Assess safety of Drug X versus Drug Y when compared in the literature.

- Article #1 – The only adverse effect that was noted to occur more frequently in the Drug X group was dry mouth. There was no difference in the incidence or severity of adverse drug reactions between the two drugs.

- Article #2 – Dry mouth was the only adverse effect noted to occur more frequently in the Drug X group compared to Drug Y.

- Article #3 – This was a case report describing 12 patients receiving Drug X that also experienced dry mouth.

• Retrieve the most current prescribing information to determine possible safety concerns.

- Dry mouth is the most frequent adverse effect associated with Drug X.

❑ Special considerations/special populations

• Establish if Drug X dosed more or less conveniently than Drug Y.

- Same dosing frequency

• Does the route of administration vary between drugs?

- Patients had more difficulty using the drug dispensing device for Drug X versus Drug Y.

• Determine if there are other potential advantages or disadvantages of Drug X versus Drug Y.

• Are there any other specific situations that may affect the population positively or negatively?

- Patients receiving Drug X who also had impaired renal function were required to have dose frequency adjustments.

❑ Cost

• Is the cost of Drug X significantly higher than Drug Y?

- Drug X is more expensive than Drug Y.

- Are there long-term cost-saving benefits of Drug X or Drug Y?
- When formulating a recommendation for a population, practitioners have fewer known specifics regarding prescription coverage, patient income, and other variables; therefore, cost does not weigh as heavily and is typically one of the final components taken into consideration when forming the recommendation.

Step 4: Categorize the Quality of Evidence

❑ Determine the level of evidence for each trial:

- Article #1 is a Level II trial with major limitation of power.
- Article #2 is a Level II trial with major limitation of power.
- Article #3 is a Level V trial with major limitations.

Article	Support/Refute	Level of Evidence	Major/Minor Limitations
1	S	II	Major-Power
2	S	II	Major-Power
3	Neither support or refute	V	Major

Figure 9.4: Summary Table of Evidence Evaluated for Example 9.3 – Population-Based Decision

Step 5: Develop a Conclusion and Recommendation (see Figure 9.4)

❑ Develop a conclusion regarding the overall efficacy based on the evidence.

- Drug X is superior in efficacy to Drug Y.

❑ Develop a conclusion regarding the overall safety based on the evidence.

- The frequency of dry mouth occurring was greater with Drug X than Drug Y.

❑ Develop a conclusion regarding any special considerations/special populations.

- The dispensing device was more difficult to use for Drug X than Drug Y.
- Patients with impaired renal function require dose frequency adjustments with Drug X.

❑ Develop a conclusion regarding the overall cost of medication specific to this population based on the following:

- Cost of Drug X versus Drug Y
  - Drug X is more expensive.
- Long-term cost benefits of either drug

❑ Assign the appropriate grade of recommendation (Figure 9.3).

❑ Develop a recommendation statement based on conclusions made and applied to this population.

❑ Example:

Recommend replacing Drug Y with Drug X on the institution's formulary for treatment of COPD for the following reasons: (Grade B Recommendation)

- Efficacy – A Level II trial shows that Drug X is superior to placebo for improving pulmonary function in COPD patients. In addition, a Level II trial shows Drug X is superior to Drug Y in improving pulmonary function in COPD patients.

- Safety – With the exception of dry mouth, there appears to be no difference in adverse drug reactions between Drug X and Drug Y.

- Special considerations/special populations – In renal impaired patients, dosing frequency adjustment is necessary with Drug X in patients with COPD. Patients who may have difficulty handling the drug dispensing device for Drug X should consider treatment with Drug Y to ensure treatment is being administered properly.

- Cost – Drug X is more expensive than Drug Y; however, there is superior improvement in pulmonary function with Drug X that justifies the additional cost. This improvement in pulmonary function may lead to fewer emergency department visits and fewer hospitalizations, therefore, lowering overall cost.

Summary

Phamacy practitioners make both individual patient and population-based decisions on a regular basis. It is imperative that they apply the 5-Step Evidence-Based Medicine Process to ensure the highest quality and most reliable evidence is being used in their clinical decision making. In addition, practitioners need to consider efficacy, safety, special considerations/special populations, and cost when making a recommendation. By taking a *less* conservative approach with individual patient decisions and a *more* conservative approach with population decisions, the pharmacy practitioner can be assured that the appropriate intervention or treatment is being recommended.

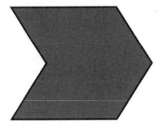

Chapter 10

Applying EBM Principles to Dietary Supplement Therapeutic Decisions

Cydney E. McQueen & Celtina K. Reinert

EBM Principles Applied to Dietary Supplements

Due to the increased use of dietary supplements over the past decade, health care providers are encountering patients who use supplements more often than they did previously. The pharmacist is frequently asked to make recommendations regarding the therapeutic use of supplements because these products are sold in many pharmacies. Just as with questions about the use of prescription drugs, the most reliable method of making recommendations is by using evidence-based medicine processes.

The same general principles of obtaining information that have already been discussed also apply to dietary supplements:

❑ When information is needed, resources are searched in the same order: tertiary, secondary, and then primary.

❑ Information found is verified in more than one source.

❑ Clinical knowledge and judgment are used along with the factual evidence, especially in making decisions about individual patient care.

When a decision must be made based on primary literature, the same 5-Step Evidence-Based Medicine Process applies to dietary supplements.

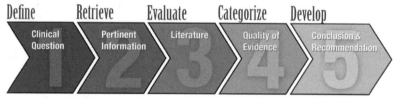

Figure 10.1: 5-Step Evidence-Based Medicine Process

Differences in 5-Step Evidence-Based Medicine Process for Dietary Supplements

If all of these principles and processes are the same, why does this book have an entire chapter on the topic of using evidence-based decision making for dietary supplements? Because *three of the EBM process steps may have crucial differences*:

❑ Step 2 – Retrieve Pertinent Information: Different search techniques and sometimes different tertiary and secondary resources must be used to ensure that retrieval of primary literature is thorough.

❑ Step 3 – Evaluate Literature: Different issues arise in the analysis of clinical trial quality.

❑ Step 5 – Develop a Conclusion and Recommendation: Different issues apply in making recommendations.

Step 1 (Define the Clinical Question) and Step 4 (Categorize the Quality of Evidence) do not differ in any way when dealing with decisions about dietary supplement therapies, *so only Steps 2, 3, and 5 are discussed here.*

Step 2 – Retrieve Pertinent Information

In drug information practice, many resources are accepted as "gold standards." That term means professionals place a very high degree of trust in the information within the reference. For instance, USP DI and AHFS Drug Information are gold standard drug information resources. Although it is always a good idea to verify information using another gold standard reference, that verification is normally done as a simple reflection of good clinical practice—pharmacists double-check everything! Errors caught by this practice are usually on the level of simple typographical or note transcription errors.

In the area of dietary supplements, no references are considered "gold standard." However, some are gaining prominence; see the table in **Figure 10.1**. Every reference published to date has flaws or expresses conclusions and recommendations that vary from other recommended resources. The same studies and case reports are often cited for conflicting or even directly opposing recommendations. In other words, the factual scientific evidence used by the authors to make a recommendation is generally the same, but the clinical interpretation and judgment allow for different conclusions.

Online Resources

Name	Approx-imate Cost	Type of Information Contained	Strengths or Advantages	Weaknesses or Disadvantages
Natural Medicine Comprehensive Database[1] www.naturaldata-base.com	$$	General	One of the most comprehensive re-sources available. Direct and to-the-point, each state-ment is referenced; hyperlinks to PubMed citations and abstracts are provided. Updated regularly and quickly when new information be-comes available. Can also research interactions, look up products by brand names, and search by medical condition.	Discussion given is very brief, and all background infor-mation necessary to make informed decisions may not be given.
Natural Standard[2] www.natural-standard.com	$$$$	General	Contains detailed information on common dietary supplements. Ex-tensive critical lit-erature review is provided in the Professional Mono-graphs. Direct links provided to PubMed abstracts. Bottom-line mono-graphs provide the same information as the Professional Monographs with-out the extensive literature review. Monographs orga-nized by medical	Smaller number of supplements dis-cussed due to de-tailed process re-quired for mono-graph develop-ment. Natural Standard is cur-rently only avail-able for purchase by university and college level aca-demic institutions, medical institu-tions such as hos-pitals, and phar-macies.

Figure 10.1: Recommended Dietary Supplement Information Resources

Name	Approx- imate Cost	Type of Information Contained	Strengths or Advantages	Weaknesses or Disadvantages
			conditions and uses. An interaction identifier is available. Supplements are indexed by brand name.	
Consumer-Lab.com[3] www.consumer-lab.com	$	Product quality, General	Independent laboratory that tests products for amount of product compared to the claimed amount, purity and tablet dissolution or disintegration. The Natural Products Encyclopedia, a general resource, is also held within this site.	Limited scope of product quality.

Print Resources

Name	Approx- imate Cost	Type of Information Contained	Strengths or Advantages	Weaknesses or Disadvantages
Natural Medicine Comprehensive Database[4], published yearly ISBN: 0978820517	$$	General	Contains monographs in the same format as online version. Also contains reference list and some brand name products and content.	Only updated once yearly, when new book is published. Dated info, time-lag. No interaction check as database.
Natural Standard Herb & Supplement Reference: Evidence-Based Clinical Reviews[5] (2005) ISBN: 0323029949	$$$	General	Same as the Professional Monographs from the online version.	Not updated as regularly as the database. Extra tools provided online are not included.

Name	Approx- imate Cost	Type of Information Contained	Strengths or Advantages	Weaknesses or Disadvantages
Natural Standard Herb & Supplement Handbook: The Clinical Bottom Line[6] (2005) ISBN: 0323029930	$	General	Provides same information as bottom-line monographs from the online version.	Not updated as regularly as the database. Extra tools provided online are not included.
Professional's Handbook of Complementary & Alternative Medicines, 3rd edition[7] (2004) ISBN: 1582552436	$	General	Monographs in a short, quick, easy-to-use format.	Minimal discussion of studies and references that monographs are based on; however, monographs are based on quality information and studies available.
Herb Contraindications & Drug Interactions, 3rd edition[8] (2001) ISBN: 1888483113	$	Interaction, Contraindications	Provides known, well-documented interactions and contraindications as well as theoretical ones. Safety-oriented resource.	Only provides interaction and contraindication information. Limited to botanical supplements only.
The 5-Minute Herb & Dietary Supplement Consult[9] (2003) ISBN: 0683302736	$$	General	Facing pages provide concise information on supplements.	Stylistically is different from other resources, but still user friendly.
Evidence-based Herbal Medicine[10] (2002) ISBN: 1560534478	$	General	Contains general monographs on just botanical supplement. Contains some info on Chinese herbs.	Limited number of monographs, limited to botanicals only.

Name	Approximate Cost	Type of Information Contained	Strengths or Advantages	Weaknesses or Disadvantages
Botanical Medicine: The Desk Reference for Major Herbal Supplements, 2nd edition[11] (2002) ISBN: 0789012669	$$	General, Pregnancy	Monographs are focused on the chemistry of the supplements. Most thorough reference available in regards to pregnancy information.	Small number of products covered, not a user-friendly resource in a clinical setting due to focus on chemistry rather than clinically important information.
Herbal Medicines, 3rd edition[12] (2007) ISBN: 0853696233	$$$	General	Partner herbal book to Dietary Supplements; same publisher, basic monograph.	British publisher, language and style differences
Dietary Supplements, 3rd edition[13] (2007) ISBN: 0853696535	$$	General	Partner dietary supplement book to Herbal Medicines; same publisher, basic monograph.	British publisher, language and style differences

Example 10.1. Different Resources, Different Answers

Three practitioners are asked to answer the question, "Can ginger be used in pregnancy and, if so, at what dose?" If each person was given a different resource to use, each one would come up with a different answer.[1,6,7]

Natural Medicines Comprehensive Database: "Possibly Safe" and "Possibly Effective;" 250 mg QID

Professional's Handbook of Complementary & Alternative Medicines: "Use in pregnancy is contraindicated"

Natural Standard Herb & Supplement Handbook: The Clinical Bottom Line: Safe and effective; 1–2 g daily in divided doses for 1–5 days

For these reasons, all information, either factual or interpreted from the facts, should be verified in a minimum of three resources. If three references have conflicting information or fail to offer a clear consensus, more resources should be used (see **Example 10.1**). Primary literature may also need to be utilized in addition to tertiary references.

Key Idea

If three references have conflicting information or fail to offer a clear consensus, more resources should be used.

Generally, tertiary resources for prescription drug products include information on interactions, adverse events and contraindications based on reports from clinical studies, post-marketing surveillance data, and sometimes published case reports.

This is true, especially if there are multiple reports of a particular problem. Most dietary supplement references do not include a caution against use in a particular disease if that caution is based only on a theoretical mechanism of action and if no clinical reports support the concern as significant. Why? Two reasons are cited: 1) there is far less clinical research on supplements than non-supplements and 2) reporting of problems with supplements is extremely low. In addition, post-marketing surveillance data are non-existent. In order to "err on the side of caution" for patient protection, practitioners need to be aware of theoretical interactions, contraindications, and potential adverse effects (see **Example 10.2**).

Example 10.2. Different Evidence, Different Recommendations

A practitioner has a diabetic patient who would like to try an herbal product for mild osteoarthritis. The two columns represent two different situations based on the evidence available.

SITUATION A	SITUATION B
References list a possible side effect of "decrease in blood sugar."	References list a possible side effect of "decrease in blood sugar."
Several clinical trials and two published case reports have *documented* patients experiencing hypoglycemic effects while using the herb.	Decrease in blood sugar is *extrapolated* from knowledge of a mechanism of action; no decreases have been reported in any clinical trials or case reports.
Recommendation: advise patient to avoid using this herb.	**Recommendation:** advise patient of possible effect, titrate up the dose of herb, and have patient monitor blood sugar more closely for 1 or 2 weeks.

In the United States, most health care practitioners depend upon Medline to electronically search for clinical trials, case reports, or other articles about many medical topics. For dietary supplement information, use of Medline alone is not sufficient to be assured of a thorough search for primary literature. Several journals that tend to publish more dietary supplement literature are not indexed in Medline. Many of them are indexed in EMBASE, another major electronic secondary resource. About one third of EMBASE-indexed journals are in common with Medline; however, EMBASE indexes more European and Asian journals. European researchers generally conduct more trials in the area of dietary supplements; therefore, they often publish in the European-based journals. Trials of traditional Oriental herbal medicines or other complementary and alternative medical therapies such as qi gong or acupuncture are often found in Asian journals.

EMBASE, in addition to other resources identified in Figure 10.1, can sometimes be found in drug information centers and/or libraries associated with academic medical centers. Some electronic resources identified are highly specialized, and locating facilities for access may be difficult. Unfortunately, many health care practitioners outside of academic or research settings will not have access to these resources, so maximizing search results via other methods becomes even more important.

Bibliographic searching involves scanning the citation list of trials, review articles, and meta-analyses to find other primary literature. This is a good method of expanding one's "reach" for searching since authors may have access to other indexing systems and, therefore, have been able to locate additional articles.

Using multiple indexing systems will not ensure a thorough search if appropriate search terms are not used. Unfortunately, identifying appropriate search terms is not a simple process. Indexing terms for supplements, especially botanical supplements, differ among indexing systems and change over time.

Common issues with indexing of dietary supplements are the following:

❑ Multiple common names

❏ Plant taxonomy changes

❏ Alternative spellings and misspellings

Multiple common names

Many supplements have multiple common names, so a thorough search should at least include the most frequently used names. For instance, co-enzyme Q_{10} is also referred to as ubiquinone. A recent search of Medline using the medical subject headings (MeSH) term, ubiquinone, returned 4,592 results, while a key-word search of "co-enzyme Q_{10}" returned 27 results, 9 of which were not contained in the MeSH term search.

With botanical supplements, a common problem is that different species may have the same common name. For instance, two unrelated plants may each be referred to as yellowroot: *Hydrastis canadensis* (usually known as goldenseal) and *Coptis chinensis* (usually known as goldthread).

Plant taxonomy changes

As in any scientific field, new knowledge changes things. Plants are sometimes reclassified and given new scientific names as botanists learn more about them. When this happens, cross-referencing of the old and new names does not always occur, so searching both is necessary. For instance, the current scientific name of black cohosh is *Actaea racemosa*, but many resources still refer to it by the former name, *Cimicifuga racemosa*. Often newer resources and electronic databases will include both current and former names.

Alternate spellings and misspellings

"Ginko" is an older spelling of "ginkgo." When searched as a keyword in Medline, "ginko" returns 10 articles that are not located using a keyword search of "ginkgo." A search of "liquorice" returns 269 articles not found when searching the American spelling of "licorice." Searching both names locates 351 articles that are not found when searching the MeSH term for the licorice family, "Glycyrrhiza."

At times, searching the same term as both a keyword and a MeSH term will provide different results. Searching with the scientific name for feverfew, *Tanacetum parthenium*, as a keyword located 28 more articles than searching *Tanacetum parthenium* as a MeSH term.

To ensure thoroughness, searches must use common names, different spellings, scientific names, and alternate scientific names. The search should be conducted via multiple methods.

Key Idea

In order to ensure a thorough search for primary literature on dietary supplements, multiple search methods and alternative terms must be used.

Step 3 – Evaluate Literature

Once the search for primary literature has led to retrieval of clinical trials, the next step is to evaluate those trials. The evaluation process is identical to the one used to analyze the quality of prescription drug products as outlined in Chapter 5: Evaluate Literature, but a few different issues arise.

A common complaint about trials of dietary supplements and other alternative therapies is that they are of poor quality. Although it is not always true, dietary supplement trials are often small or moderate in size and have significant design limitations. First, limited funding is available for research in this area. Government agencies such as the National Institute of Health's National Center for Complementary and Alternative Medicine are providing more funding for large, professionally managed studies. Many trials are still conducted on a shoestring budget by practitioners who are not properly trained in how to conduct research. These disadvantages can sometimes affect the overall quality of study design. Another problem is that the researchers may be experts in their field of practice, but lack expertise in use of supplements or natural therapies. Because there may be multiple problems with these trials, evaluation of evidence quality and systematic decision making becomes even more important.

Several trial limitations common to dietary supplement trials have been identified:

- ❑ Power and/or sample size
- ❑ Biostatistics
- ❑ Product/dose
- ❑ Blinding
- ❑ Outcome measures

Power and/or sample size

The smaller sample size often observed with dietary supplement trials is primarily an issue of funding. Many supplement manufacturers interested in conducting research are simply not large or profitable enough to afford to enroll a substantial number of patients to confidently determine differences between groups.

Biostatistics

This limitation could also be related to lack of funding (i.e., not being able to afford statistician consultation). In addition, researchers could lack expertise. Today, it is very easy for the average person to buy and use statistical programs to analyze data ... and very easy to tell the computer to use the wrong test!

Product/dose

The best dose of a dietary supplement is frequently not known and doses for trials are based on common usage, which may or may not be an effective dose (see **Example 10.3**).

Example 10.3. Different Preparations, Different Unknowns

There are multiple species of echinacea, three of which are used medicinally. To date, it is unknown which of the three species is the most effective, which plant parts are best used, or what is the best type of preparation (whole herb, pressed juice, extract). These "unknowns" may help to explain the highly variable results seen in efficacy trials.

A common complaint by medical herbalists or naturopaths is that researchers often use inappropriate products or preparations. For instance, a study of glucosamine hydrochloride does nothing to answer the clinical question about whether glucosamine sulfate relieves symptoms of osteoarthritis (see **Example 10.4**).

Example 10.4. Different Products, Different Results[14,15]

Several years ago, while headlines were trumpeting the results of a study saying, "garlic has no effect on lipid levels," natural medicine practitioners were replying, "of course it didn't work!" Researchers had chosen to use a garlic oil supplement that was heat processed—the high temperatures destroyed all allicin content, the ingredient believed to be the one responsible for any positive effects.

Another complaint that has been truer in the past than recently is the use of insufficient doses of comparator drugs. For instance, many of the early St. John's wort studies for depression used only 75 mg of imipramine, a starting dose that would generally be subtherapeutic for most patients.[16] These studies produced results unfairly biased in favor of the dietary supplement.

Blinding

Blinding difficulties are usually an issue with botanical supplements rather than with the non-botanical supplements such as melatonin and glucosamine. Many of these plant products have very distinctive tastes or smells, and it can be impossible to make identical placebos. For instance, the herb valerian, used for anxiety, sleep, or muscle cramps and spasms, is quite pungent and identifiable.

Another type of blinding difficulty is when a supplement has a very distinctive side effect that allows it to be distinguished from the placebo. For instance, fenugreek, a supplement tested for effects on lowering blood sugar, has been reported to cause a "maple syrup" smell in the urine of many who use it.

Outcome measures

Another limitation often seen in supplement trials is the use of non-standard outcome measures (i.e., measures not commonly used and accepted for monitoring symptoms of a disease state). For instance, if researchers create a questionnaire about symptoms of depression rather than using a validated measurement such as the Hamilton Depression Scale, the results would not be widely accepted by other medical practitioners.

These areas are not the only ones in which methodological limitations might be found. They are simply the areas in which it is most common to find problems when critiquing trials of dietary supplement therapies.

Step 5 – Develop a Conclusion and Recommendation

This step of the process uses the same principles as non-dietary supplement recommendations described in Chapter 7: Develop a Conclusion and Recommendation; however, some different factors need to be considered.

Patient autonomy is a greater issue. Many patients who use supplements place a higher priority on making decisions about their health and treatment. Although health care providers have the duty to provide accurate information and their own recommendations to a patient, the right to self-determination must be respected.

Key Idea

Health care providers have the duty to provide accurate information and recommendations to patients; however, patient autonomy must be respected.

Another concern to keep in mind is product quality. Patients and practitioners don't generally have to think about quality with prescription drugs, but contamination, adulteration, and differing amounts of claimed active ingredients can be a serious issue with some supplements. When making recommendations about using a specific type of supplement, health care providers should also help guide patients to a high-quality product. Brands recommended by health care professionals should either be participating in a quality seal program or be tested by a third-party laboratory. At the very least, products should be made by a large reputable company, preferably one that also produces prescription or OTC drugs (see the table in **Figure 10.2**).

Patients and care providers should work together to evaluate both the known and possible risks and benefits of any particular supplement when making a therapeutic decision. Some questions to consider are as follows:

❑ Is this product safe for use?

- Do data show it is generally safe and non-toxic? Is there information on dose-related toxicities? Consider if the patient has any specific contraindications to use of the drug, or if he/she is on any medications that interact with the supplement.

❑ Is this product effective for use?

- If the product is not effective, how much, if any, harm will be done by not treating the patient's condition? Also, consider the extent of effectiveness. For example, a patient who needs to lower cholesterol by 20 mg/dL might be a good candidate for a supplement in addition to lifestyle changes, while a patient who needs lowering by 120 mg/dL is not a good candidate.

❑ Is this condition self-treatable and able to be self-monitored?

- Some conditions cannot be considered self-treatable because of the potential for worsening of the disease. An example would be depression due to the risk of suicide.

Method of Assurance	Definition	Examples	Comments
Quality Seal Programs	If a manufacturer agrees to abide by standards and quality control measures as set by the offering company or institution, it is allowed to display a seal on supplement labeling as an indicator that the product meets certain requirements.	DSVP – Dietary Supplement Verification Program from the United States Pharmacopeia, the standard-setting organization for United States drug manufacturers.[17] TruLabel – from the Natural Products Association.[18]	All quality seal programs are voluntary and may have different standards of quality. Mandatory for NPA member companies that manufacture their own labeled products.
Ratings from a Third-Party Laboratory	A third-party laboratory purchases supplements "off the shelf" and tests them for quality.	Consumer Lab.com[19] Consumer Reports from Consumers Union	ConsumerLab also offers a quality seal program. Only reviews products occasionally, so information in magazines may be out of date. Some information from the Natural Medicines Comprehensive Database is available on the Consumer Reports web site.
Reputable Manufacturer	A large, reputable company that also produces prescription or non-prescription drugs.	Glaxo-Smith Kline – produces prescription products such as Amoxil® and Zantac®, and also the dietary supplement, Alluna®.[20]	The rationale behind this assurance method is that these companies are required to follow Good Manufacturing Practices (GMPs) for the drug products they produce. If they already have such strict quality control procedures in place for some products, they are more likely to use quality control measures for other products.

Figure 10.2: Product Quality

❑ Is this a high quality product?

- For example, is it in a quality seal program or has it been evaluated by a third-party program?

❑ Do the benefits outweigh the risks of using the product?

❑ Is there another product (prescription, OTC, or dietary supplement) that would work better for this patient and this condition?

Summary

The process of evidence-based decision making for dietary supplements is the same as for prescription drugs, although a few differences apply:

❑ Primary literature retrieval search techniques require more thought and planning, and perhaps more "legwork," since more indexing systems must be used.

❑ Literature evaluation generally requires consideration of different, and sometimes more, limitations than prescription drug studies.

❑ Additional considerations need to be addressed when making recommendations.

References

1. Jellin JM, Gregory PJ, Batz F, et al., eds. Natural Medicines Comprehensive Database [database online]. Stockton, CA: Therapeutic Research Faculty. Available at www.naturaldatabase.com.

2. Basch E, Ulbricht C, eds. Natural Standard [database online]. Cambridge, MA; Natural Standard. Available at www.naturalstandard.com.

3. Cooperman T, Obermeyer W, eds. ConsumerLab.com. [database online]. White Plains, NY: ConsumerLab.com, LLC. Available at www.consumer lab.com.

4. Jellin JM, Gregory PJ, Batz F, et al., eds. *Pharmacist's Letter/Prescriber's Letter Natural Medicines Comprehensive Da-*

tabase. 9th ed. Stockton, CA: Therapeutic Research Faculty; 2007.

5. Ulbricht CE, Basch EM, eds. *Natural Standard Herb & Supplement Reference: Evidence-Based Clinical Reviews.* St. Louis, MO: Mosby, Inc.; 2005.

6. Basch EM, Ulbricht CE, eds. *Natural Standard Herb & Supplement Handbook: The Clinical Bottom Line.* St. Louis, MO: Mosby, Inc.; 2004.

7. Fetrow CW, Avila JR, eds. *Professional's Handbook of Complementary & Alternative Medicines.* 3rd ed. Philadelphia, PA: Lippincott; 2004.

8. Brinker F. *Herb Contraindications & Drug Interactions.* 3rd ed. Sandy, OR: Eclectic Medical Publications; 2001.

9. Fugh-Berman A. *The 5-Minute Herb & Dietary Supplement Consult.* Philadelphia, PA: Lippincott, Williams & Wilkins; 2003.

10. Rotblatt M, Ziment I, eds. *Evidence-Based Herbal Medicine.* Philadelphia, PA: Hanley & Belfus; 2002.

11. McKenna DJ, Jones K, Hughes K. *Botanical Medicine: The Desk References for Major Herbal Supplements.* 2nd ed. New York, NY: The Haworth Herbal Press, Inc; 2002.

12. Barnes J, Anderson LA, Phillipson JD. *Herbal Medicines.* 3rd ed. London, UK: Pharmaceutical Press; 2007.

13. Mason P. *Dietary Supplements.* 3rd ed. London, UK: Pharmaceutical Press; 2007.

14. Berthold HK, Sudhop T, Bergmann K. Effect of a garlic oil preparation on serum lipoproteins and cholesterol metabolism: a randomized controlled trial. *JAMA.* 1998; 279(23):1900–1902.

15. Lawson L. Effect of garlic on serum lipids. *JAMA.* 1998; 280(18):1568.

16. Vorbach EU, Hubner WD, Arnoldt KH. Effectiveness and tolerance of the hypericum extract LI 160 in comparison with imipramine: randomized double-blind study with 135 outpatients. *J Geriatric Psychiat Neurol.* 1994; 7(Suppl 1):S19–23.

17. United States Pharmacopeia. USP Verified Dietary Supplements [database online]. Available at: http://www.usp.org/USPVerified/dietarySupplements. Accessed August 2007.

18. Natural Products Association (formerly National Nutritional Foods Association) TruLabel Program [online database]. Available at: http://www.naturalproductsassoc.org/site/PageServer?pagename=ic_bg_trulabel. Accessed August 2007.

19. ConsumerLab. The CL Seal. Available at: http://www.consumerlab.com/seal.asp. Accessed August 2007.

20. GlaxoSmithKline. Product list. Available at: http://www.gsk.com. Accessed May 2008.

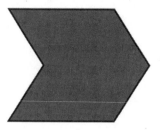

Glossary of Evidence-Based Medicine Terms

Absolute Risk Reduction (ARR) – The absolute difference between the rates of outcomes between two groups. For example, let us assume that a study evaluating the efficacy of two different medications in preventing secondary myocardial infarctions (MI) in patients with known risks was performed using two active treatments. For patients receiving Treatment A, 15% experienced a secondary MI compared to only 5% of patients receiving Treatment B who experienced a secondary MI. The ARR for Treatment B is (A – B) or 0.15 – 0.05, which equals 0.1 or 10%. This value may be more useful in evaluating the true impact of a therapy versus relying on the relative decrease in risk (see *Relative Risk Reduction* and *Number Needed to Treat*).

Alpha Level (α) – The probability of making a Type I error (see *Type I Error*). In hypothesis testing, this value is also the p-value threshold for a result to be statistically significant. Statistical significance is noted to occur when the p-value is less than the α-level.

Alternative Hypothesis – The study hypothesis that is usually the exact opposite of the null hypothesis (see *Null Hypothesis*). In medical research, the alternative hypothesis usually states that there *is* a difference between study groups. For example, if the null hypothesis is that A = B, then the alternative hypothesis could be A ≠ B. There can also be multiple alternative hypotheses. Using the previous example, the multiple alternative hypotheses could be set up as 1) A > B and 2) B > A.

Applicability – How well the results of a clinical study will fit into "real world" practice settings. Also referred to as relevance.

Bayesian Analysis – An analysis beginning with a specific probability that then incorporates new data or information resulting in a revised probability (prior probability and posterior probability, respectively).

Beta Level (β) – The probability of making a Type II error (see *Type II Error*). This value is related to the "power" of a study, which equals $1 - \beta$.

Bias – An error credited to the investigative team or subject/patient that provides results different from the true results and leads to a potentially wrong interpretation of the overall study results.

Binomial – Data that has only two outcomes.

Blinding – A study design method utilized to neutralize the potential for biased study results based on inaccurate reports from patients, health care providers, and study investigators. Classifications of blinding include:

Open Label – No blinding exists. Patients, health care providers, and study investigators all know what treatment is being given at all times.

Single Blinding – The patient is unaware of what treatment arm he/she is assigned. This reduces the potential that a patient will report a positive or negative outcome based upon a predisposed "feeling" of how well a treatment works or does not work (i.e., placebo effect).

Double Blinding – The patient, health care provider, and study investigators are unaware of what treatment arm the patient has been assigned. This blinding method reduces the bias of the patient, health care provider, and study investigator using predisposed "feelings" when assessing how a study treatment is working during a clinical trial. This method is particularly useful because the health care provider must remain objective in the management of the patient's disease state through a clinical trial.

Triple Blinding – The patient, health care provider, study investigator, and an outcomes assessor are all blinded. In this scenario, the health care provider is utilized to provide only data, and a distinctly different individual evaluates the data to provide the outcome conclusion. This individual remains blinded to the assigned treatment arm in order to maintain objectivity when completing outcomes assessments. A good example of this situation is when a patient is being treated for a fungal infection in the lungs. The health care provider and/or study investigator monitors the patient through the clinical trial. However, the individual who provides the final determination of clinical success or failure would be a radiologist examining the patient's chest x-rays. Using a very specific set of criteria, this unbiased, blinded third party makes an objective determination of clinical success or failure.

Triple blinding is a much less common approach to clinical trial design than double blinding. However, in clinical trials that rely on more "qualitative" results (e.g., x-rays) rather than numerical laboratory tests, the use of an independent third party to determine clinical success or failure can lead to more scientifically sound results by eliminating the inter-rater variability present when using multiple health care providers who might have multiple opinions of clinical success or failure.

Quadruple Blinding – Very rarely reported, the patient, health care provider, study investigator, outcomes assessor, and data analyst are all blinded to the patient's assigned treatment group.

Case-Control Study – An observational study design method commonly used when studying rare disease states or outcomes, such as a rare side effect. A case is identified with the outcome that the investigator is studying. Control patients (those lacking the outcome being studied) are then matched to the case as closely as possible, usually using age, gender, race, etc. Then, the investigator retrospectively evaluates the case and control histories to identify any characteristics associated with the case group and *not* associated with the control group. This method is prone to multiple biases; caution should be used when making any conclusions based on results of this trial design.

Case Report – A description of an individual patient with a disease or outcome that is of interest. There is no control group.

Case Series – A consecutive collection of patients (case reports) with the same disease that is treated in the same manner. There is no control group.

Clinical Guidelines – See *Practice Guideline*.

Clinical Significance – Results from a clinical study that show a difference large enough to justify changing the way a practitioner would usually treat patients. The results reveal practical as well as statistical importance.

Cohort – A group of study subjects who share a common exposure or characteristic. A cohort study commonly compares two large groups of individuals—those who have received (but not assigned) a specific intervention and those who have not. The two groups are usually observed prospectively over time to evaluate the long-term outcomes.

Cointervention – A treatment or treatments that are not the primary study intervention (concomitant treatments) that may actually have an effect that will bias the study results.

Confidence Interval (CI) – The range or interval of data in which the "true" result is thought to exist with a given percentage of "confidence." The CI is related to the alpha level set for statistical significance. For example, if the α-level is set at 0.05, then the CI is 95% (calculated as $1 - 0.05$). A 95% CI simply means that, with 95% confidence, the study results indicate the true value measured lies within the reported range. However, there is a residual 5% chance that the true value lies outside of the calculated range, which prevents a CI from being a conclusive estimate.

Confounding Variables – An unknown factor (e.g., patient characteristic, environmental cause, changes in medical practices over time) that could have contributed to the effect seen in a clinical trial, unrelated to the intervention. Researchers aim to eliminate confounding variables so that the results of a clinical trial can provide as much conclusive evidence of a measured benefit as possible. Proper study design is the best way to minimize confounding variables. Randomization of study subjects to the treatment groups is a common method of minimizing confounding variables.

Consecutive Sample – A sample of patients, all of whom were potentially eligible, enrolled, and seen over a period of time.

Control Group – A group of patients that do not receive the study intervention. They may receive a placebo or other active treatment that is often times the "gold standard."

Convenience Sample – A patient or group of patients that are selected at the convenience of the investigator or were available at a convenient place or time.

Correlation – The degree of relationship noted between two or more different variables or observations.

Correlation Coefficient – A numerical expression (between -1.0 to 1.0) of the degree of relationship noted between two or more different variables

Cost Analysis – When two or more strategies are analyzed but only the costs are compared, not costs and expected outcomes.

Cost Benefit Analysis – When two or more strategies undergo an economic analysis that includes both costs and consequences articulated in monetary terms.

Cost-Effectiveness Analysis – When two or more strategies undergo an economic analysis that includes both costs and consequences articulated in natural units such as cost per life saved.

Cost Minimization Analysis – When two or more strategies undergo an economic analysis where the consequences for each are the same, thus the only issue is their relative costs.

Crossover Trial – A type of study design in which study participants receive both treatments. By "crossing over" to the comparison treatment arm, each participant serves as its own control group. When evaluating the outcomes of these studies, it is important to ensure that there was an appropriate length of "washout" before the participants crossed over into the second treatment group. Too short of a washout period can allow residual pharmacodynamic effects of the first treatment to influence the results of the second treatment, which could give misleading results.

Cross-Sectional Trial – A type of study design that evaluates a defined population at a single point in time. The national census survey is a good example of a cross-sectional trial.

Decision Analysis – A systematic process using a mathematical model that includes various identified components to make the best possible clinical decision.

Decision Tree – An analytical tool used to express the various components that go into a decision analysis.

Dependent Variable – The outcome variable in a study. This variable is affected by changes in the independent variable.

Descriptive Statistics – Statistics that summarize, tabulate, and organize data to describe study observations or measurements.

Effect Size – The difference in outcomes between the study group and the control group divided by a measurement of variance such as the standard deviation.

Effectiveness – The measurement of a treatment's "true" impact on a particular disease state in a "realistic" setting. The *effectiveness* of a treatment can differ greatly from its own estimation of *efficacy* (see *Efficacy*). The effectiveness of a treatment is influenced by a number of factors, including the frequency of administration required to achieve a therapeutic effect, the administration route, the treatment's cost to the patient, the treatment's side effect profile, the patient's perceived benefit from the treatment, and the treatment's social acceptance. Many of these factors result in patient non-compliance to therapy. Sometimes, a *less efficacious* treatment can be *more effective* at treating or maintaining a disease state when studied in the "real world" setting.

Efficacy – The measurement of a treatment's "potential" impact on a particular disease state in a "perfect" setting. Efficacy is usually determined in very controlled situations that do not always have the same extraneous influences that exist when studying a treatment's "true" *effectiveness* (see *Effectiveness*). Large phase III clinical trials are commonly used to determine a treatment's efficacy. The FDA generally approves medications based on efficacy, not effectiveness, data in addition to other considerations such as safety. However, once approved and released to the general population, a medication's *potential efficacy* can be very different from its resultant *true effectiveness*.

Endpoint – Health event(s) or outcome(s) that signify completion or termination from a trial such as death or loss to follow-up.

Equivalence Study – A study designed to show equivalence between treatments in safety, efficacy, or other parameters. Also called non-superiority studies.

Event Rate – Proportion of patients in the experimental group (experimental event rate) and/or control group (control event rate) that a predefined event is observed.

Follow-up – A process to determine the outcome in every patient who participated in a clinical trial.

Frequential Statistics – The statistical method of using frequencies of an outcome to determine probabilities or odds of an outcome occurring. This method does not take into account past experience with the outcome's probability, such as a Bayesian Analysis method. Frequential statistics are currently the most common method used to evaluate the results of controlled clinical trials.

Generalizability – The capability to take the results generated by a study and generalize to a larger and similar population of patients.

Gold Standard – A well accepted therapeutic approach considered the standard of practice for a particular disease state.

Hawthorne Effect – The phenomenon where a patient's performance is improved because he/she is aware that his/her behavior is being observed.

Hazard Ratio – The weighted relative risk over the time of the entire study.

Incidence – Number of new cases of a specific disease over a set time.

Independent Variable – The treatment variable that is assumed to have some effect on the outcome or dependent variable.

Inferential Statistics – The process of making conclusions based on the results from a sample of the population of interest.

Intention-to-Treat (ITT) Analysis – A method of statistical analysis that maintains randomization by incorporating all patients in their originally assigned groups during data analysis, regardless of whether the patient finished the study. This also includes patients lost to followup. This type of analysis can more accurately depict the clinical significance of a studied treatment. For example, if the researchers only analyzed the outcomes of the patients who finished the trial, then the safety and benefits of a treatment could be over- or underestimated. ITT Analysis can be very complex in its methods, but a study that utilizes this analysis generally is considered to have more validity in its results.

Interobserver Variability – Variation in outcome results by different observers.

Interval Data – Continuous data scales with known, equal distance between each interval (e.g., blood pressure, blood glucose).

Interventional Study Design – A study design in which subjects receive a treatment (or intervention) they would not otherwise receive and the effect on a particular outcome is observed.

Intraobserver Variability – Variation in outcome results by the same observer during repeat testing.

Likert-type Scales – An instrument used by study investigators to capture a patient's rating of his/her response such as pain; a scale that measures extremes of attitudes or feelings, generally using 3 to 9 possible values such as no pain, mild pain, moderate pain, and severe pain.

Lost to Follow-up – The inability to determine the outcome of a patient who participated in a clinical trial.

Matching – An intentional process to create similar study and comparative groups based on patient characteristics. This is seen primarily in observational case-control studies to help substantiate that differences in results between the groups are due to the study intervention of interest.

Mean – A measurement of central tendency or, in other words, the arithmetic average.

Meta-Analysis – A statistical method of compiling results from various studies to obtain a pooled result representing "new data." The goal of a meta-analysis is to increase statistical power through an increase in the pooled sample size. Meta-analyses are commonly used to clarify the roles of treatment in specific clinical situations that have conflicting results. A meta-analysis can also answer new questions not previously reported in original manuscripts, but this generally requires access to the original study data that is not often readily available. It is important to note that a meta-analysis cannot convert a poorly designed study into a well-designed study; the quality of the results in a meta-analysis is entirely dependent upon the quality of data going into the analysis.

N of 1 trial – Type of crossover trial in which a single patient or small numbers of patients serve as their own control and receive alternating courses of treatment over a specific period of time.

Nominal Data – Categorical data that cannot be ranked (e.g., yes/no, male/female, hair color, eye color).

Non-Dinomial – Data that is not limited to two outcomes (also non-binomial).

Non-Parametric Distribution – Data that, when graphed, fall into a non-normal distribution and do not form a bell-shaped curve.

Non-Parametric Tests – Statistical tests that do not assume a normal distribution of data. These statistical tests are used when the data is skewed, but can also be used for non-skewed data.

Null Hypothesis – The "baseline" hypothesis that is generally thought to be true but has not been proven. In medical research, the null hypothesis usually states that there is no difference between study groups. There can only be one null hypothesis in a given study. The directive of the study is to either *reject* the null hypothesis OR *refuse to reject* the null hypothesis. Note that *refusing to reject* the null hypothesis is not the same as *accepting* the null hypothesis to be true.

Number Needed to Harm (NNH) – The number of patients who need to receive a treatment before 1 patient is "harmed" that would not have occurred if all of those patients received the comparison treatment. NNH is calculated from the reciprocal of the absolute percent difference in incident rates of a specific adverse event between two study groups. For example, if Treatment A is associated with a 5% incidence of rash, and Treatment B is associated with a 2.5% incidence of rash, then the NNH for Treatment A would equal 1 / (0.05–0.025). This equals 40 patients who need to be treated with Treatment A before 1 patient gets a rash that would NOT have otherwise occurred had all 40 patients received Treatment B. Ideally, the *higher* the NNH is for a treatment, the better.

Number Needed to Treat (NNT) – The number of patients who need to receive a treatment before 1 patient reports a positive outcome that would not have occurred if all of those patients received the comparison treatment. NNT is also equivalent to the reciprocal of the absolute risk reduction (1 / ARR) (see *Absolute Risk Reduction*). For example, if Treatment A is associated with a 30-day mortality rate of 20%, and Treatment B is associated with a 30-day mortality rate of 10%, then the NNT for Treatment A would equal 1 / (0.2 – 0.1). This equals 10 patients who need to be treated with Treatment A to prevent 1 death at 30 days, which would NOT have otherwise occurred had all 10 patients received Treatment B. Ideally, the *lower* the NNT is for a treatment, the better. Generally, medications that are used to actively treat a disease state (e.g., antibiotics in treating pneumonia) have lower NNTs than medications that are used to prevent the development of a particular disease state (e.g., aspirin in preventing stroke).

Observational Study Design – A study in which no intervention is made on the subjects; observations are made on naturally occurring events.

Odds – A ratio of probability comparing occurrence to nonoccurrence of a particular event.

Odds Ratio – The ratio of the odds of exposure in case patients divided by the odds of exposure in control patients. This is commonly reported in case-control studies and prospective cohort studies.

Operator-Dependent – A phenomenon where the results of a test are dependent upon the specific skills of the person conducting the test.

Ordinal Data – Data that can be ranked in specific order. The intervals between data points are not equal distance (e.g., Likert pain scale).

Outcome – The result(s) associated with a medical intervention on a subject or patient. Measurements for the outcome are generally established prior to conducting the trial. Investigators often establish *primary outcome(s)* and *secondary outcome(s)*. The primary outcome(s) is generally used to calculate the required sample size to meet a set power, thus assuring that a difference between study groups is identified, if one truly exists.

P-Value – The probability that random chance is the source of the observed difference between two test variables and is not related to the treatment being studied. In other words, the smaller the p-value, the more likely the observed difference is due to something other than random chance. If the p-value is less than the pre-established α-level, then the p-value is considered "statistically significant" (see *Alpha Level* and *Type I Error*).

Parallel Study Design – Study design in which two or more groups receive treatment simultaneously and are compared.

Parametric Distribution – Data that, when graphed, fall into a normal distribution of a bell-shaped curve.

Parametric Tests – Statistical tests that assume the data is normally distributed (i.e., bell curve).

Per Protocol Analysis – A method of statistical analysis where the investigators analyze the outcomes of only those patients who completed the trial. Patients lost to followup are not included. This type of analysis can result in overestimating or underestimating the safety and benefit of a treatment.

PICO – A strategy used to define the clinical question that takes into consideration the patient(s), intervention(s), comparison(s), and outcome(s).

Point Estimate – The estimated value from the study sample of participants. In a representative sample, the point estimate is considered the *best* estimate of a population.

Power – The ability of a study to detect a statistically significant difference between two groups when a difference truly exists. The lower the power a study has, the more likely it is to find no statistically significant differences when, in reality, a difference truly does exist—which is considered a "false negative" (see *Type II Error*). Power is directly affected by sample size, variance, and the magnitude of difference between means. The determination of a study's true power can be very complex, but in its most simplistic form power can be calculated as $1 - \beta$ (see *Beta Level*).

Practice Guideline – A systematically developed series of statements providing guidance and direction for a practitioner regarding the treatment of a patient's specific disease. These guidelines are developed by either consensus of experts, evidence-based medicine principles, or a combination of both.

Prevalence – The frequency of a disease determined by the number of patients in a population who have a specific disease at a given time.

Prospective Study Design – A study design in which observations are made as the data is collected and groups are followed forward in time.

Qualitative Research – Research offering insights into behavioral, social, and emotional events associated with health care. Subjective in nature.

Quantitative Research – Research involving the testing of specific hypotheses focusing on variables that will provide numbers and measurements suitable for statistical analysis. Objective in nature.

Randomized Controlled Study – A study design where subjects or patients are randomly assigned to an intervention or a control group. The randomization is performed to assure that each subject or patient has an equal opportunity of ending up in either group(s). When randomization is successful, each study group is similar in characteristics and demographics.

Ratio Data – Continuous data scales with known, equal distance between each interval; they contain a non-arbitrary, absolute zero (i.e., no negative numbers).

Relative Risk – The ratio of the risk of an outcome in a treatment group divided by the risk of the outcome in the control group. In a controlled, clinical trial the risk of an outcome is the same as the probability or incidence. The relative risk of an outcome is also our "natural" interpretation of risk ratios. This is commonly the number we consider when describing a treatment to be "_____ *times as likely*" to have a particular outcome.

Relative Risk Reduction (RRR) – The relative difference between the rates of outcomes between two groups. For example, let us assume that a study evaluating the efficacy of two different treatments in preventing secondary myocardial infarctions (MI) in patients with known risks was performed using two active treatments. For patients receiving Treatment A, 15% experienced a secondary MI compared to only 5% of patients receiving Treatment B who experienced a secondary MI. The RRR for Treatment B is calculated as (A – B) / A or (0.15 – 0.05) / 0.15, which equals 0.667 or 66.7%. The RRR of a treatment generally inflates the true benefit of a treatment, which is why RRR is the most commonly reported number in the news media. Absolute risk reduction and number needed to treat may be better measures to use when comparing two treatment options (see *Absolute Risk Reduction* and *Number Needed to Treat*).

Reliability – The ability of a test or process to provide the same results when repeated with similar conditions.

Retrospective Study Design – A study design in which observations are made looking back in time at data that already exists.

Sample – A part of the population that is selected to participate in the study.

Sensitivity – A test's ability to identify a true-positive rate such as the presence of a specific disease.

Sensitivity Analysis – An analytical procedure used to verify what effects would occur to the results from changing input variables.

Specificity – A test's ability to identify a true-negative rate such as the non-presence of a specific disease.

Standard Deviation – A measurement of the spread from the mean. A large variance reflects a large spread from the mean or, in other words, a large standard deviation.

Statistical Inference – See *Inferential Statistics*.

Statistical Significance – A measure of confidence concerning an observed difference between study groups and whether that difference is due to the study treatment or just chance alone.

Stratified Randomization – A method to ensure balance between different study groups regarding important factors that may have an effect on the outcome.

Surrogate Endpoint – A measurable (and usually quantifiable) test result that makes inferences towards an actual clinical outcome. Surrogate endpoints are commonly used in clinical trials to measure the efficacy of a treatment using a smaller sample size in a shorter amount of time. Also, surrogate endpoints are commonly used in treatments that are in the early stages of development. As experience is gained with a new treatment, the use of surrogate endpoints is replaced with actual clinical outcomes data. A surrogate endpoint also gives patients and health care professionals a biomarker useful for monitoring the ongoing efficacy of a therapy, such as with antihypertensive agents and the blood pressure measurement. Surrogate endpoints *must* have a strong correlation with a clinical outcome in order to be useful in making inferences towards the actual patient outcome. For example, measuring blood pressure is a good surrogate marker that has substantial clinical data correlating it to the risk of cardiovascular mortality.

Systematic Review – A formal evaluation involving a pertinent literature search and critical literature appraisal to answer a defined clinical question. No "new data" is created.

Treatment Effect – A measurement used to express the results of comparative clinical studies. These measurements include Absolute Relative Risk, Relative Risk Reduction, Odds Ratio, Number Needed to Treat, and Effect Size.

Type I Error – Falsely determining that a statistically significant difference between two study variables exists when, in reality, no difference truly exists (i.e., false positive). The probability of a Type I error occurring is related to the alpha level set by investigators (see *Alpha Level*).

Type II Error – Falsely determining that no statistically significant difference between two study variables exists when, in reality, a difference truly does exist (i.e., false negative). The probability of a Type II error occurring is related to the beta level set by investigators (see *Beta Level*).

Validity – The measure of confidence one has that the results are true, believable, and free from bias. Validity can also represent the level of confidence that a measurement accurately represents what it is supposed to measure.

Variable – Anything that can take on different values such as an outcome measurement, characteristic of a group, risk factor, etc.

Variance – A measurement of the spread of values around the mean. Also see *Standard Deviation*.

Washout Period – The period of time required for the pharmacological effect of a treatment to end once the treatment has been discontinued. In crossover clinical trials, an adequate washout period should be maintained between treatment phases. Failure to do this can result in the pharmacological effect being carried over to the alternate treatment phase, thus confounding the results.

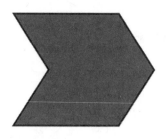

Evidence-Based Medicine Tool Kit

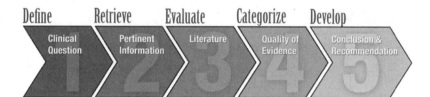

5-Step Evidence-Based Medicine Process Diagram

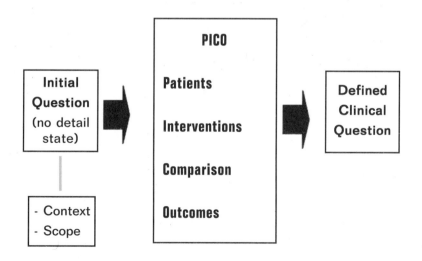

Define	Retrieve	Evaluate	Categorize	Develop
Clinical Question	Pertinent Information	Literature	Quality of Evidence	Conclusion & Recommendation
1	2	3	4	5

Define the Clinical Question

Initial Question (no detail state)

- Context
- Scope

PICO

Patients

Interventions

Comparison

Outcomes

Defined Clinical Question

Ten Major Considerations

Article Title:_____

Level: (circle one)   I   II   III IV V

Limitations: (circle one)   Major   Minor

MAJOR CONSIDERATIONS *with Justifications for Each*		S	L
Power set/met?	yes/no		
Dosage/treatment regimen appropriate?	yes/no		
Length of study appropriate to show effect?	yes/no		
Inclusion criteria adequate?	yes/no		
Exclusion criteria adequate?	yes/no		
Blinding present?	yes/no		
Randomization resulted in similar groups?	yes/no		
Biostatistical tests appropriate for type of data analyzed?	yes/no		
Measurement(s) standard/validated/accepted practice?	yes/no		
Author's conclusions are supported by the results?	yes/no		

Levels of Evidence to Categorize Quality of Evidence

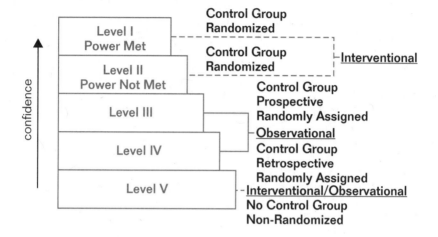

Summary Table of Evidence Evaluated

Clinical Question - _____

Article	Outcome	Level of Evidence	Major Limitations

Grading Tool to Determine Strength of Recommendation

GRADE A
Level I Trials

_____
_____
_____

GRADE B
Level II Trials

_____
_____
_____

GRADE C
Levels III, IV,
& V Trials

_____
_____
_____

Recommendation Format

THE RECOMMENDATION STATEMENT

JUSTIFICATION IN A BULLET FORMAT
- Efficacy
- Safety
- Other special considerations/populations
- Cost

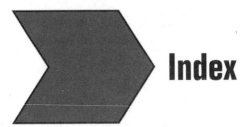

Index